LENS:
The Low Energy
Neurofeedback System

LENS: The Low Energy Neurofeedback System has been co-published simultaneously as *Journal of Neurotherapy*, Volume 10, Numbers 2/3 2006.

Monographic Separates from the *Journal of Neurotherapy*

For additional information on these and other Haworth Press titles, including descriptions, tables of contents, reviews, and prices, use the QuickSearch catalog at http://www.HaworthPress.com.

LENS: The Low Energy Neurofeedback System, edited by D. Corydon Hammond, PhD (Vol. 10, No. 2/3, 2006). *Examines the research, development, and clinical applications of the revolutionary LENS method of brain wave feedback.*

Forensic Applications of QEEG and Neurotherapy, edited by James R. Evans, PhD (Vol. 9, No. 3, 2005). *Examines new and potentially very useful ways of verifying, preventing, and treating criminal behaviors; provides many valuable references for clinicians and researchers.*

New Developments in Blood Flow Hemoencephalography, edited by Tim Tinius, PhD (Vol. 8, No. 3, 2004). *Introduces the technique of operant conditioning of brain blood flow via feedback of information on oxygenation and brain temperature obtained by non-invasive instrumentation.*

Quantitative Electroencephalographic Analysis (QEEG) Databases for Neurotherapy: Description, Validation, and Application, edited by Joel F. Lubar, PhD (Vol. 7, No. 3/4, 2003). *Provides cutting-edge information on quantitative electroencephalographic analysis (QEEG), the most popular QEEG databases, and QEEG's applications in medicine.*

LENS:
The Low Energy
Neurofeedback System

D. Corydon Hammond, PhD

Editor

LENS: The Low Energy Neurofeedback System has been co-published simultaneously as *Journal of Neurotherapy*, Volume 10, Numbers 2/3 2006.

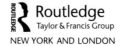

Routledge
Taylor & Francis Group
NEW YORK AND LONDON

First published 2006 by The Haworth Press, Inc.

Published 2016 by Routledge
711 Third Avenue, New York, NY 10017
2 Park Square, Milton Park, Abingdon, Oxon OX14 4RN

Routledge is an imprint of the Taylor & Francis Group, an informa business

First issued in hardback 2015

LENS: The Low Energy Neurofeedback System has been co-published simultaneously as *Journal of Neurotherapy*, Volume 10, Numbers 2/3 2006.

Library of Congress Cataloging-in-Publication Data

LENS : the Low Energy Neurofeedback System / D. Corydon Hammond, editor.
      p. / cm.
   "Simultaneously co-published as Journal of neurotherapy, volume 10, no. 2/3, 2006."
   Includes bibliographical references and index.
   ISBN 978-0-7890-3568-4 (pbk)
   ISBN 978-1-138-13602-1 (hbk)
   Biofeedback training. 2. Electroencephalography. I. Hammond, D. Corydon. II. Title: Low Energy Neurofeedback System.
   [DNLM: 1. Biofeeback (Psychology)–methods. 2. Biofeedback (Psychology)–instrumentation. 3. Nervous System Diseases–
therapy.
W1 JO795EM v.10 no. 2/3 2006 / WL 103 L573 2006]
RC489.B53L46 2006
615.8'51–dc22
                                                                      2006030006

LENS:
The Low Energy
Neurofeedback System

CONTENTS

ABOUT THE EDITOR

D. Corydon Hammond, PhD, ABPH, ECNS, QEEG-D, BCIA-EEG, is a licensed Psychologist and full Professor in Physical Medicine & Rehabilitation, University of Utah School of Medicine. He is a past President and Fellow of the International Society for Neuronal Regulation, a past President and Fellow of the American Society of Clinical Hypnosis, a Fellow of the Society for Clinical & Experimental Hypnosis, and a Fellow of the Academy of Family Psychology. Dr. Hammond is board certified in EEG, Quantitative EEG brain mapping, and neurophysiology from the EEG and Clinical Neuroscience Society, and also in QEEG from the Quantitative EEG Certification Board. He is certified in neurofeedback by the Biofeedback Certification Institute of America, and is a Diplomate of the American Board of Psychological Hypnosis and the American Board of Family Psychology. He has served as a board member of the Neurofeedback Division of the Association for Applied Psychophysiology and Biofeedback. He has published 9 previous books (winning 3 best book of the year awards from professional societies) and more than 100 professional journal articles, reviews or chapters in books. He is an Associate Editor of the *Journal of Neurotherapy* and on the editorial boards of several other journals. He co-chaired the Task Force on Methodology and Empirically Supported Treatments in the areas of biofeedback and neurofeedback. He has served as Chair of a joint ISNR/ AAPB/BCIA Standards Committee, and as Chair of the Public Information Committee and the Professional Education Committees of ISNR. He is the primary author of the standards for the use of QEEG in neurofeedback. In 2005 he received the Joel F. Lubar Award from ISNR for services to the society and the field of neurotherapy.

Preface

LOW ENERGY NEUROFEEDBACK SYSTEM: NEW IDEAS, TREATMENT, AND METHODS

My experience has led me to conclude that most patients/clients and professionals do not like learning about new treatment methods, especially those diseases and diagnoses related to brain functioning. For patients and clients, they are comfortable with simple information provided on many occasions and through visual media or reading. This media information is simple, easy to understand and presented repetitively. People become comfortable with the information and when they are comfortable with the information, they begin to believe that the information is true and not question the basis of the information. For professionals, a paradigm shift in how to treat a person with a diagnosis after they leave school/training is difficult when they learn that the treatment involves electronic machines and computers. For example, they are comfortable with the treatment methods of psychotherapy, medication and relaxation as they are simpler to understand, conceptualize and implement, and most importantly, the professional does not have to learn computer analysis or brain wave patterns. Professionals are trained with methods that seem intuitive and practical, but when they encounter a new treatment, they often use a criterion that is much higher than the criterion for currently accepted treatment models or like our clients/patients, they are comfortable with the information and do not question the assumptions. Often this culminates in a view of "no change" and we will do what we have always done because it is just too difficult to conceptualize or explain a new treatment; and besides psychotherapy and medication are good for many problems and diagnosis.

As you read this publication of the *Journal of Neurotherapy* on a treatment called Low Energy Neurofeedback System or LENS, please remain open to new ideas and technology that can help our clients and patients. I purposely did not use the word "new" as this treatment method was in development for 15 years. (In our quickly changing society, the word new is often innovative and positive, but in the helping professions, "new" is met with skepticism and questions.) I remember many years ago when Dr. Ochs discussed the combination of lights and EEG used during feedback and I was interested from the point of how one could use this treatment to decrease the number of sessions. This volume of the *Journal of Neurotherapy* provides our readers with an in depth look at LENS, provides a history of the treatment, and describes the potential for this technology to impact the field of neurofeedback or EEG biofeedback. This treatment has the potential to be another tool in our toolbox of helping patients with brain related diseases and diagnosis.

Tim Tinius, PhD
Editor
Journal of Neurotherapy

[Haworth co-indexing entry note]: "Preface." Tinius, Tim. Co-published simultaneously in *Journal of Neurotherapy* (The Haworth Medical Press, an imprint of The Haworth Press, Inc.) Vol. 10, No. 2/3, 2006, p. xvii; and: *LENS: The Low Energy Neurofeedback System* (ed: D. Corydon Hammond) The Haworth Medical Press, an imprint of The Haworth Press, Inc., 2006, p. xi. Single or multiple copies of this article are available for a fee from The Haworth Document Delivery Service [1-800-HAWORTH, 9:00 a.m. - 5:00 p.m. (EST). E-mail address: docdelivery@haworthpress.com].

Introduction

D. Corydon Hammond, PhD

This volume introduces the reader to a unique, innovative neurofeedback/neurotherapy technology called the Low Energy Neurofeedback System (LENS). The LENS treatment method has gradually evolved over the past 16 years primarily through the innovations of Len Ochs, PhD. In this volume you will read about the LENS, its historical evolution, and its application in the treatment of a variety of diagnostic problems.

By way of introduction, let me offer a personal perspective. In the 1990s I listened to meeting presentations by Len Ochs and felt extremely puzzled. He often expressed his belief that neurofeedback clinicians were overtraining their patients and that many patients did not need 30-minute long training sessions. In fact, he said that sometimes even 10 seconds of treatment might be too much. At that point in time the previous version of the LENS used photic stimulation in association with the EEG biofeedback. In my clinical work I often used a neurofeedback system that had similarities to the LENS in its use of photic stimulation. However, despite using what seemed to be relatively similar equipment, I simply could not resonate with Len Ochs' statements about over-stimulating patients by having lengthy treatment sessions. My training sessions with patients were 30 minutes long and yet, in the majority of cases, my patients reported significant improvements in their symptoms following this traditional neurofeedback. Finally, I dismissed what Dr. Ochs was saying. It simply did not fit with my own clinical experiences.

Soon after the beginning of the new century I came to understand the reason for the disparity between our clinical experiences. Len Ochs asked the Lawrence Livermore Labs to do an analysis of his equipment. They discovered, much to everyone's surprise, that the extremely weak photic stimulation associated with his treatment was not the operative factor. The analysis determined that there was a unique element with the system–an exceptionally tiny electromagnetic pulse was being delivered down the electrode wires to head of the patients. The timing of the electromagnetic pulses was determined by the way in which the lights were timed to flash in relationship to the dominant brainwave pattern of the patient. The LENS system now became comprehensible to me. It was understandable that some patients could feel over-stimulated by this treatment–the LENS training was completely different from other neurofeedback systems. A very weak electromagnetic signal was influencing the brain, which could understandably have the potential influence of over-stimulating someone if they received too large a dose.

Research has found that the far far stronger electromagnetic field emitted by a cell phone can have potential negative effects on EEG brain patterns. For instance, Kramarenko and Tan (2003) found that after 20 to 40 seconds of cell phone usage, slow wave activity (2.5-6.0 Hz) appeared in the contralateral frontal and temporal areas. These slow waves, lasting for about one second, reoccurred every 15 to 20 seconds at the same recording electrodes. After

---

D. Corydon Hammond is Professor, Physical Medicine and Rehabilitation, University of Utah School of Medicine, 30 North 1900 East, Salt Lake City, UT 84132.

[Haworth co-indexing entry note]: "Introduction." Hammond, D. Corydon. Co-published simultaneously in *Journal of Neurotherapy* (The Haworth Medical Press, an imprint of The Haworth Press, Inc.) Vol. 10, No. 2/3, 2006, pp. 1-4; and: *LENS: The Low Energy Neurofeedback System* (ed: D. Corydon Hammond) The Haworth Medical Press, an imprint of The Haworth Press, Inc., 2006, pp. 1-4. Single or multiple copies of this article are available for a fee from The Haworth Document Delivery Service [1-800-HAWORTH, 9:00 a.m. - 5:00 p.m. (EST). E-mail address: docdelivery@haworthpress.com].

Available online at http://jn.haworthpress.com
doi:10.1300/J184v10n02_01

the cell phone was turned off the slow wave activity progressively disappeared, and local changes decreased and disappeared after 15 to 20 minutes. They found similar changes in children, but the slow waves had higher amplitude and appeared earlier in children (10 to 20 seconds) than adults. They found that their frequency was lower (1.0-2.5 Hz), occurred at shorter intervals, and had a longer duration. Research thus suggests that cellular phones may reversibly influence the human brain, inducing abnormal slow waves in the EEG of awake persons. In contrast, as you will read in this volume, a few seconds of exposure to the much weaker electromagnetic fields from LENS has a therapeutic effect of reducing high amplitude slow activity in the EEG. The difference seems to be that (a) the electromagnetic signal is far weaker, and (b) it is individualized and updated 16 times each second so that it remains at a frequency that is consistently faster than the patient's dominant EEG frequency.

Having learned about the Lawrence Livermore Lab analysis, I could now comprehend how the LENS training operated and, therefore, no longer believed that Len Ochs must be from another galaxy far, far way. Nonetheless, I was still troubled by one other contingency. Dr. Ochs talked about a few patients feeling side effects associated with LENS treatment. Prior to understanding the operative mechanism in LENS treatment, patients often received 5, 10, or even 20 minutes of treatment. This could certainly cause some patients to feel over-stimulated or fatigued. Even though I observed that refinements in both the equipment and clinical procedures were being made, I was still concerned about even a small percent of my patients having a side effect where they felt "wired or tired," even though this rarely lasted for more than one day.

Another reservation stemmed from my lingering doubts about how sessions could produce therapeutic changes when they only consisted of the delivery of a few seconds of stimulation. Even though I saw encouraging research appearing on the use of LENS treatment with fibromyalgia (Donaldson, Sella, & Mueller, 1998; Mueller, Donaldson, Nelson, & Layman, 2001) and traumatic brain injuries (Schoenberger, Schiflett, Esty, Ochs, & Matheis, 2001), I was still skeptical. The professor part of me won-

dered how much of a placebo response was involved. It certainly seemed possible that positive expectancies could be fostered by clinicians, leading to placebo responses. Consequently I simply continued using more traditional neurofeedback which I knew was usually effective.

An experience then challenged my thinking. Two years before editing this volume, I was a participant on a panel at a professional society meeting with Dr. Stephen Larsen, a decade long colleague of Dr. Ochs. Stephen was talking about his experiences in using LENS with animals. For example, he described a dog that had been hit by a car, began having seizures, and had become aggressive. After a small number of sessions the seizures ceased and the dog's former pleasant demeanor returned. As I heard these case reports of animals, in contrast to my patients, it seemed very hard to imagine that a dog who was having electrodes placed on his head was reasoning at some level, "Gosh, this is going to make me feel better, quit biting people, and stop having seizures!" I decided to investigate LENS more seriously. I first reread the published research reports and then talked with therapists in three different countries who had been applying LENS clinically. I was favorably impressed and obtained training from Len Ochs.

Although I had casually known Len Ochs for many years, as I studied hours of videotapes of him teaching and then spent two days being individually tutored by him, I was deeply impressed by his personal characteristics. In a field focused on technology, he emphasizes the importance of the therapeutic relationship and creating rapport. He exudes a kindness and caring. What was perhaps most impressive was the fact that despite more than three decades of clinical experience and the creative innovations he has brought to this field, he remains modest and refreshingly honest. He candidly admits how much is still not known about LENS treatment, how it achieves its effects, and the fact that LENS treatment does not succeed with all patients.

In spite of his unpretentiousness and the fact that LENS research is still in its infancy, I am convinced that Len Ochs has created a technology that has great therapeutic potential. It is for this reason that I decided to edit this volume. LENS is unique in that it does not require the patient to "work" during neurofeedback. The fact that the patient is not required to have the impulse control, attention, or stamina to concentrate for significant periods on a computer screen can be particularly appealing. These factors open up new possibilities for the treatment of patients who are very young, oppositional, seriously autistic or disabled, minimally able to cooperate, and even for the humanitarian treatment of animals with brain-based disorders.

In over 30 years of clinical practice as a psychologist I have been cautious about new treatments that lacked research support. In particular I have been wary of any therapeutic approach that presented itself as being the "one true light"–a panacea for all the various clinical conditions we find in our patients. This has also been my stance since entering the field of neurofeedback fourteen years ago. I have tried to remain open to learning from different individuals and approaches within the field. Many experienced professionals have things to offer and a single approach to neurotherapy is unlikely to produce positive outcomes with everyone. I have studied the research on iatrogenic effects that began being published in the 1960s and 1970s. This research informs us that when a therapist follows a unitary approach to treatment and fails to individualize therapy, this is one of the primary factors associated with producing adverse and negative effects. Thus I have remained eclectic in my approach to the practice of neurofeedback. I value still having my traditional neurofeedback tools available to me, and I prize the addition of LENS to my therapeutic armamentarium.

My own clinical experience with LENS suggests that it is not always superior to other types of neurofeedback–but what approach within psychology or psychiatry is always successful? With many patients, however, I have found that LENS treatment produces unusually rapid, even startling symptomatic improvement. In the same way that we teach our patients, I believe that it is likewise important for clinicians to not engage in dichotomous reasoning, either-or thinking. Our treatment options are not limited to a choice between either using the LENS or reliance on more traditional neurofeedback approaches. Many clinicians will use LENS as well as other neurofeedback modalities, sometimes with the same patient. Thus when I have a

patient who has experienced 8 to 10 LENS sessions and he or she does not display some symptomatic improvements, I will often add traditional neurofeedback and reduce the dosage of LENS training. This decision stems from two factors. First, Len Ochs often says, "Less is more." By this he means, as he explains in his paper, that sometimes a lack of symptomatic improvement may stem from the patient receiving too large an amount of stimulation/feedback. Therefore, I may reduce the amount of LENS input from perhaps six seconds (one second at each of six electrode sites) to only two seconds, and spend the remainder of the session doing more traditional neurofeedback. The second rationale for adding another modality is something that I have already emphasized–nothing works for all patients. In still other cases I have seen the rapid symptomatic improvements that commonly occur with LENS in the first 10 to 20 sessions, but then progress may have slowed, but further improvements are still desired. In such a case, other traditional neurofeedback modalities may also be added to the therapy.

This volume provides a valuable introduction to LENS. It begins with an extensive overview by Len Ochs. His introduction includes information about the historical evolution of his equipment, theoretical background, and practical information about the clinical use of LENS. The next contribution is a very well done, double-blind, placebo-controlled research study with fibromyalgia. What may surprise our readers is that this study by Kravitz and his colleagues did not produce the hoped for results. It is nonetheless included (with the encouragement of Dr. Ochs) because we can learn as much from publishing negative results as from positive outcomes. We should not be afraid to publish such studies. Two commentary articles follow the fibromyalgia study. They are illuminating in helping us understand the reasons that the Kravitz study did not produce positive results. The first commentary by Len Ochs elaborates details that were unknown at the time of the study about the operative mechanism in the feedback, and about the excessive dosage level that was being administered. The second commentary by Mary Lee Esty, a co-author of the Kravitz research study, discusses the multi-causal nature of fibromyalgia and the fact that no single modality, such as neurofeedback, can hope to address all of the etiologic factors. The Esty commentary will prove enlightening for all clinicians working with fibromyalgia, and it will encourage more thorough pre-treatment assessment and a broader conceptualization of interventions that may be helpful with this condition.

The next contribution is from the Stone Mountain Center, led by Dr. Stephen Larsen. This large clinical research paper presents a case series of 100 patients treated with the Low Energy Neurofeedback System. The systematic symptom ratings provide impressive documentation of the rapid treatment effects that commonly occur with LENS training and their relationship to reductions in EEG amplitudes. This study is particularly encouraging because it demonstrates the effectiveness of LENS with a very broad range of symptoms in only 20 sessions. The next clinical paper is by Dr. Curtis Cripe, who presents three case reports on his work with the LENS in the treatment of serious neurodevelopmental and learning disability problems. Although LENS treatment is only one component within his treatment model, Dr. Cripe describes the invaluable role that he has found it to play. The final contribution is by Dr. Stephen Larson and his co-workers on the use of LENS training with animals that are experiencing neuro-behavioral problems.

We do not yet have enough controlled research in the field of neurofeedback in general, including with regard to LENS treatment. This volume, and the few studies that have already been published, simply provide an encouraging foundation from which to proceed. For me, however, one of the most exciting aspects of LENS treatment is that by its very nature it lends itself to conducting double-blinded placebo controlled experiments with both animals and humans–something that holds tremendous promise for advancing the field of neurofeedback in gaining acceptance by the evidence-based medical, psychological, neuroscience, and academic communities. Such studies are already underway and we look forward to learning more from their results.

REFERENCES

Donaldson, C. C. S., Sella, G. E., & Mueller, H. H. (1998). Fibromyalgia: A retrospective study of 252 consecutive referrals. *Canadian Journal of Clinical Medicine, 5* (6), 116-127.

Kramarenko, A. V., & Tan, U. (2003). Effects of high-frequency electromagnetic fields on human EEG: A brain mapping study. *International Journal of Neuroscience, 113* (7), 1007-1019.

Mueller, H. H., Donaldson, C. C. S., Nelson, D. V., & Layman, M. (2001). Treatment of fibromyalgia incorporating EEG-driven stimulation: A clinical outcomes study. *Journal of Clinical Psychology, 57* (7), 933-952.

Schoenberger, N. E., Shiflett, S. C., Esty, M. L., Ochs, L., & Matheis, R. J. (2001). Flexyx neurotherapy system in the treatment of traumatic brain injury: An initial evaluation. *Journal of Head Trauma Rehabilitation, 16* (3), 260-274.

doi:10.1300/J184v10n02_01

The Low Energy Neurofeedback System (LENS):
Theory, Background, and Introduction

Len Ochs, PhD

SUMMARY. This article presents the concepts, operations, and history of the Low Energy Neurofeedback System (LENS) approach as they are now known and as it has evolved over the past 16 years. The conceptual bases and practical operating principles as described are quite different from those in traditional neurofeedback. The LENS, as a behavioral neurofeedback application, often provides the same qualitative outcome as that in traditional neurofeedback, with reduced treatment time. doi:10.1300/J184v10n02_02 *[Article copies available for a fee from The Haworth Document Delivery Service: 1-800-HAWORTH. E-mail address: <docdelivery@haworthpress.com> Website: <http://www.HaworthPress.com> © 2006 by The Haworth Press, Inc. All rights reserved.]*

KEYWORDS. Neurofeedback, EEG biofeedback, biofeedback, neurotherapy, LENS, low energy neurofeedback system, EEG, brain stimulation

INTRODUCTION

The Low Energy Neurofeedback System (LENS) is an EEG biofeedback system used in clinical applications and research in the treatment of central nervous system functioning. It is unique in the field of neurofeedback in that instead of only displaying information on a computer screen to assist the patient in conditioning healthier brainwave patterns, the LENS uses weak electromagnetic signals as a carrier wave for the feedback to assist in reorganizing brain physiology. The following describes the rationale for the LENS system, as well as subsequent discoveries. Also presented are some suggestions for future research and practical application of the LENS technology.

Evolution of LENS and Relevant Concepts

The major implication of this paper is that both the physically and psychologically traumatized brain has demonstrated vastly greater capacity for recovery than has previously been appreciated. Secondarily, the LENS appears to help the traumatized person achieve clearly increased performance in relatively short periods of time, with a quite non-invasive, low technology procedure. On the other hand, other kinds of EEG biofeedback may be just as effective as the LENS under some conditions. Although no claims are being made here that the LENS is better than any other form of treatment, it is, however quite different from other neurofeedback modalities, as well as from other

Len Ochs is affiliated with Ochs Labs, Sebastopol, CA.

Address correspondence to: Len Ochs, 8151 Elphick Lane, Sebastopol, CA 94596 (E-mail: lochs@earthlink. net).

[Haworth co-indexing entry note]: "The Low Energy Neurofeedback System (LENS): Theory, Background, and Introduction." Ochs, Len. Co-published simultaneously in *Journal of Neurotherapy* (The Haworth Medical Press, an imprint of The Haworth Press, Inc.) Vol. 10, No. 2/3, 2006, pp. 5-39; and: *LENS: The Low Energy Neurofeedback System* (ed: D. Corydon Hammond) The Haworth Medical Press, an imprint of The Haworth Press, Inc., 2006, pp. 5-39. Single or multiple copies of this article are available for a fee from The Haworth Document Delivery Service [1-800-HAWORTH, 9:00 a.m. - 5:00 p.m. (EST). E-mail address: docdelivery@haworthpress.com].

neurostimulation techniques such as audio/visual stimulation and particularly transcranial magnetic stimulation, where the intensities used are thousands of times stronger than LENS uses. Lastly, there appears to be no basic science yet revealed to help understand the phenomena described here, thus creating a new area of inquiry in the neuro-behavioral sciences.

The following section is presented for historical purposes to outline the order and context in which the significant components in the development of the LENS were observed including: a description of the instrumentation; the means of measuring and controlling the feedback intensity; the problems and benefits observed in the development of this system; and treatment management problems and how they evolved, particularly with regard to different populations.

History. During the summer of 1990, Harold L. Russell, PhD of Galveston, Texas, telephoned Len Ochs, PhD in Concord, California. He asked Ochs to develop a device which provided fixed-frequency photic stimulation. His interest was based upon the work of Marion Diamond, PhD (1988) in her work on the effects of environmental stimulation on cortical complexity in rats. Russell (Carter & Russell, 1981, 1984, 1993) had experimented with exposing school children with performance problems and high inter-test variability to daily, 20-minute repeated cycles of 10 Hz, for one minute, then 18 Hz for a minute, for six weeks. Russell used bright red flashing lights inside improvised welder's goggles. His idea was to use the flashing lights to stimulate the brains of the school children.

It was my impression that any simple fixed-frequency stimulation would be an inefficient way to provide the desired stimulation to alter brainwave activity. The degree to which a person's EEG (electroencephalographic activity) is influenced by external (e.g., photic) stimulation depends on many factors, including their dominant brainwave frequency from moment-to-moment, and the intensity and frequency of the stimulus used. Although the intensity and frequency of a fixed stimulation frequency could influence the EEG, another factor that might have bearing on entrainability of the EEG is the size of the difference, at any moment, between the stimulation frequency and the predominant energy of the EEG, in which lies the dominant frequency. The dominant frequency is the frequency at that moment at a spot on the person's head which is stronger than any other frequency. With that as a hypothesis, it seemed appropriate to suggest that a treatment approach might be to tie the stimulation frequency to the dominant, or peak, EEG frequency.

Since from 1 in 4,000 children and about 1 in 20,000 adults are estimated to be photosensitive (Quirk et al., 1995), and thus vulnerable to experiencing a seizure with photic stimulation, this could occasionally present severe problems. Photo-hypersensitivity refers to the reactivity to light that is strong enough to elicit convulsions–whether the person is epileptic or not. If, for instance, the person were to have a seizure–whether from epilepsy or the stimulation evoking a photohypersensitive seizure–the frequency of that seizure would become the dominant frequency. In other words, if the stimulation frequency equaled the dominant frequency, the stimulation would further stimulate any pre-existing seizure. Fortunately this could be dealt with easily by programming the software to prevent the software from ever being equal to the dominant frequency. An example of how to do this was to define the stimulation frequency as some percentage of the dominant frequency. It was anticipated that this strategy would begin to displace and disperse some of the energy of any seizure activity to other non-seizure brainwave frequencies. Fortunately, setting the stimulation frequency to some percentage greater than 100% of the dominant EEG might satisfy those in the neurofeedback community (Lubar, 1985) advocating for increasing EEG frequencies for enhanced cognitive control. Further, using a percentage less than 100% of the dominant frequency might satisfy those advocating decreasing EEG frequencies for enhancing emotional integrity and decreasing chemical dependence (Peniston & Kulkosky, 1991). Russell agreed to pay for the programming of the original software according to this conception. Hence, the software was programmed into devices that would be called electroencephalographic entrainment feedback (EEF).

The original EEF software was designed to link together the J&J I-330 EEG module 201 (and afterward the J&J I-400), and the Synetic Systems Synergizer (Seattle, Washington), a light-and-sound generation device which fit inside an IBM-clone computer through software know as BOS, a DOS-based interpreted platform developed by William Stuart, of Bainbridge Island, Washington. As originally conceived, the software was to allow the Synergizer card to set the flash frequency of the lights inside some welder-type goggles, and to continuously reset their speed as the dominant EEG frequency of the person's brain changed on a moment-to-moment basis. The software also set and reset the frequency of binaural auditory tones coming through ear phones, in the same way it set the light frequency. The feedback might pulsate at 105% of the dominant frequency during one 10-second period, then 95% of the dominant frequency during the next, and alternate between the two conditions. The software never let the flash frequency equal the dominant frequency.

The initial system, funded by Russell's AVS group, involved many features that have now been discarded, while the current software now includes many features that were not yet conceived. Discarded features central to the original conception were: the necessary use of visible light feedback, the use of sound feedback, the use of fixed time limits for changing offsets, the use of the same size offsets from the dominant frequency, the necessary use of offsets, the necessary use of alternating offsets, and the necessary use of offsets of arbitrary sizes.

New features include the generation of the feedback signal from within the EEG (the electroencephalograph) device itself, as well as the ability to control the feedback, using the J&J I-330 C2 family of EEGs. The use of the J&J I-330 C2 permitted the portable use of the system from a suitable desktop or notebook computer.

It is important to note that there were many technical inadequacies of the first generation EEF system. Yet the results from this technically "inadequate" system appeared to be better than any other treatment for closed-head trauma. Interestingly, the results were not quite as good when the more technically sophisticated second generation system was introduced. This led those involved to try to duplicate some of the inadequacies of the original system. The major required change was to retard the feedback, which was produced much more rapidly in the replacement unit for the I-330 C2. We had to introduce a time lag between the occurrence of any EEG event and the feedback tied to its occurrence. The critical learning from this experiment was that technical precision does not necessarily lead to clinical efficacy. The current use of the LENS employs extremely weak intensities of feedback and does involve the patient's own EEG driving the feedback, but does not involve any conscious participation or even positive intention.

Differences Between the LENS and Traditional Neurofeedback

The following statements reflect the current status of the EEG biofeedback field at this time.

1. The field of EEG biofeedback or neurofeedback is relatively new. There are relatively few studies with chronic conditions, controlled or otherwise, that offer understandings of what will work, under what conditions, to what extent, and with what time, physical, and monetary costs.
2. Each of the various kinds of EEG biofeedback involves its own set of rituals, with relatively little analysis of what alternatives might be used.
3. None of the forms of EEG biofeedback appear to have ever cured a progressive condition such as Alzheimer's, multiple sclerosis, Parkinsonism, or dementia. However, they probably have increased functioning and quality of life for many people in the earliest stages of any of these diseases, perhaps for at least several years and when applied properly.
4. Each form of EEG biofeedback seems to complement and enhance the effects of all of the others, as well as other forms of therapy.
5. Based on interviews with former patients of nearly each form of EEG biofeedback, each approach seems roughly comparable in effects, no matter how inexpensive or how expensive the treatment was, with some specific differences from treatment-to-treatment to be defined with later research.
6. Nearly all forms of EEG biofeedback work with easy cases and become more

cumbersome and delicate (with satisfactory outcomes) with complex cases, but appear nevertheless at their clinical efficacy limit with the current technologies because of technical problems of managing coherence and other issues.

7. Finally, while each form of EEG biofeedback may appear scientific, the application of each is probably more of a physiologically-based art than science at this stage of the game. Even so, all of the forms of EEG biofeedback seem to offer provocative and interesting hope for many who have been declared to be at the end of their options for improvement.

The LENS differs from traditional EEG biofeedback in that the LENS does not require the person to understand the meaning of, or laboriously attend for a half hour to the feedback in order to influence their brainwave activity and benefit from the treatment. No attentional, discrimination, prolonged stillness, or learning demands are placed on the individual. In addition, the LENS uses a somewhat different conceptual approach to selection of which EEG sites to train. Traditional neurofeedback uses protocols based on either symptoms or on abnormalities found in QEEG brain maps, with both approaches often utilizing only a limited number of electrode sites for training. In contrast, the LENS treatment is also guided by a topographic EEG map, but one which prioritizes electrode site abnormalities based on both EEG amplitude and EEG variability. Unlike other neurofeedback approaches, LENS treatment is then administered at all 19 (or more) electrode sites. Treatment consists of the delivery of a tiny electromagnetic field carrying the feedback signal down the electrode wires for only one second at each of the chosen electrode sites during every session. This input stimulation varies from moment-to-moment, updated 16 times per second based on the dominant EEG frequency changes. Generally between one and seven of the ordinary electrode sites are treated during each session.

Finally, central to the application of LENS treatment is the concept of patient reactivity/ sensitivity and the response of the patient's nervous system. We adapt the duration of stimulation, session frequency, and degree to which the stimulus is offset from the dominant EEG frequency to the patient's reactivity, and closely related to their vitality and degree of symptom suppression.

The LENS may be used as a tool to use in a treatment context with other EEG biofeedback or neurofeedback modalities or as a single solution to several problems. The LENS is being studied as a potential treatment of adults and children with CNS-mediated disorders in the USA, Australia, Canada, Germany and Mexico. It has been shown to produce rapid resolution of difficult cognitive, mood, anxiety, clarity, energy, physical movement and pain problems when compared with more traditional forms of psychotherapy or medication treatment. No efficacy comparisons are offered in relation to other forms of EEG biofeedback, or neurofeedback, since no comparative studies have been undertaken.

It is important to note that the LENS does not require the patient's attention, focus, orienting toward feedback, home practice of self-regulation techniques, or, indeed, any conscious participation in any self-regulatory activity (except showing up and not removing the electrodes from the head). The LENS appears to operate on the basis of the biophysical properties of the feedback signals themselves, on the tissues of the brain and related structures such as the vascular system. In addition to not requiring attention, focus, and attention toward feedback, the LENS approach, tolerates gross movement and artifact without reducing efficacy, or inappropriately rewarding maladaptive behavior or physiological reactions.

Feedback signals of different intensities, frequencies, and wave form shapes appear to have different clinical effects. There are only the beginnings of sophisticated research into the properties of the OchsLabs system. It is still too early to draw any conclusions about the mechanisms or properties of the systems used. The LENS can be used with extremely hyperactive patients and still maintain apparent efficacy. The LENS feedback exposures can be as short as one second per session for the appropriate patient and still have apparent efficacy, which means that it demands relatively little cooperation from the patient.

Benefits of LENS

The LENS appears to: (a) increase ease of functioning; (b) increase clarity of functioning; (c) reduce the amplitude and variability (including spiking) of the EEG activity across the 1-40 Hz spectrum at each of the standard 10-20 electrode sites when there is some amplitude and variability to start with; (d) increase the amplitude and variability of the EEG when there is too little variability sometimes to show the full extent of the pathology, before it diminishes the amplitude and variability; (e) reduce or alleviate central nervous system problems as described below; (f) allow new information (psychotherapy, counseling, education, relationship-specific information from a spouse or co-worker, etc.) to be recognized, taken in, used and remembered much more easily without interference or defensiveness.

The LENS appears to shorten the treatment times required for the improvement of some serious cognitive, mood, energy, pain, and motor control impairments. The LENS also appears to offer patients previously considered untreatable a new option for remediation of symptoms. Based on experience with both EEG biofeedback research, and the use of pulsating lights and other energy fields in neurological examinations to study seizure activity, it is hypothesized that the mechanism of action involves altering the person's maladaptive inhibitory neurotransmitter activity. The LENS has been declared a "minimal-risk" device by several independent human subject review boards (IRBs).

Improved functioning has been observed for those patients receiving the LENS treatment who had plateaued in their recovery from motor paralysis and CNS-mediated cognitive and mood impairment after mechanical and psychological trauma. Reported improvements have persisted since data collection was begun in 1994 (and even earlier with antecedent systems).

Improvement has been reported in most of the subjects (N = 2500, in approximately 90,000 sessions as of 2005) who have been treated with the LENS. When the subjects for this research and treatment have fallen within the areas that are known to be particularly treatable such as mild traumatic brain injury, fibro-myalgia, and explosive autism, the success rate has reached over 80%. The more the patient's history has been complicated by lifelong problems preceded by an intergenerational history of problems in parents and grandparents, and when the patient's problems have been numerous and complex, it is much more complicated to judge the efficacy of this approach; thus, the "success rate" may drop precipitously.

Side effects from the use of the LENS have been similar to those that result from any change in situation (biofeedback, meditation, moving a household, body work; i.e., disruptive upon over stimulation) but transient and not involving any organ system damage or dysfunction. The three most common side effects when there has been over stimulation have been fatigue, anxiety or hyperactivity, and no improvement in clinical symptoms. All of these situations resolved themselves, usually within a few hours or days, by temporary withdrawal from treatment and decreased exposure to feedback.

Optimal Kinds of Cases. The LENS appears to have its best effects for: (a) mild traumatic brain injury if the person was formerly high functioning; (b) the diffuse pain of fibromyalgia and its associated fatigue and mental fogginess, but leaving untouched any underlying myofascial pain for conventional treatment; and (c) explosive behavior, regardless of its cause, whether it is in an adult, a non-autistic child, or an autistic child.

More Difficult But Positive Cases. The LENS has been shown in uncontrolled, anecdotal experience, to produce less consistent, less reliable, and more difficult-to-obtain–but nevertheless still positive, results in cases of: (a) autism: more sociability, greater affection, verbal skill, more grace and balance; (b) trauma from childhood sexual or physical abuse, work, and war stress; (c) clinical depression secondary to anxiety disorder; (d) bipolar disorder secondary to anxiety disorder; (e) alcohol and cocaine addiction: less craving, less defensiveness and depression; (f) childhood schizophrenia and Asperger's syndrome: less fear, greater independence and achievement; less compliance (not to be equated with oppositional), greater independence, less fearfulness and anxiety, and more self-direction; (g) some types of chronic fatigue syndrome: greater energy and clarity;

(h) attention-deficit disorders; (i) physical head injury symptoms from moderate to severe. In the latter case positive outcomes were found in clinical research that was conducted under Office of Alternative Medicine-National Institutes of Health Grant to determine the efficacy of the LENS on reducing cognitive deficits among people suffering from closed head injuries (Schoenberger, Shiflett, Esty, Ochs, & Matheis, 2001).

It is important to note that while clinical improvement has been noted in all of the conditions cited above, the course of treatment with the LENS alone was often inelegant, cumbersome, involving trial and error and clinical skill. The reasons for the complexity of treatment are reasonably well understood. However we still have not evolved treatment protocols to solve the treatment complexity problems and make them as apparently successful and easy in the discrete conditions that were noted above as areas of application where the best effects have been achieved.

METHODOLOGY AND DISCUSSION

The LENS Treatment Process

The LENS works by continuously monitoring EEG activity and then uses these readings to determine the frequency of very small electromagnetic fields that are "offset" several cycles per second (hertz) faster than the patient's dominant brainwave. This feedback stimulus input is then delivered down electrode wires at generally seven or fewer electrode sites in the course of a treatment session, for only one second per site. This input is much weaker than what the brain receives from holding a cell phone to one's ear.

How can non-perceivable feedback to the brain that is of such minimal magnitude still be influential? While the mechanism of how this happens remains to be determined, it is clear from both the documented effects of these feedback signals on the amplitudes and variability of brainwaves, that (a) this feedback is being processed by the brain, and (b) the impact of these signals, when used correctly, can improve people's functioning in their own experience and the experience of others who observe them.

While these effects are clear to the professionals who use the LENS, it remains the job for controlled, double-blind, randomized studies to demonstrate these effects to others. It also remains for basic research to describe the mechanisms that allow these effects to take place, as well as the variables which minimize and maximize the effects.

The current the LENS process involves:

1. Assessing the sensitivity, reactivity, fragility, hardiness, and prior history of problematic symptoms that are no longer present. This is done with a simple questionnaire found in the Appendix B.
2. An assessment looking at the following:

   a. The relative proportion of different frequency band activity within the raw EEG. If there is more delta amplitude, then it is likely there may be an acquired problem such as head injury. If alpha is predominant then there may be more of a pervasive developmental issue such as ADD with genetic influences.
   b. The clinical reaction to a standard dose of stimulation feedback. There is no substitute to putting a toe in the water, experiencing some of the feedback, and then looking at what happens over the next twenty-four hours. Then, despite theoretical ideas about the appropriateness of the dose, the person may find that the dose in that administration is just right, or too much. Signs that it may be too much are that the person is profoundly fatigued, or restless and overly energized, both of which usually disappear within twenty-four hours.
   c. Assessment of which offset frequency from the dominant frequency is most efficacious at which to present stimulation.
   d. If the prospective client appears reasonably sturdy, an offset evaluation is performed to assess these factors.
   e. If the person appears from the evaluation to be vulnerable to over stimulation, a much shorter and less intense evaluation is done, giving all the in-

formation above except a suggestion about which offset to use. The offset frequency is then presumed to be 20 Hz faster than the dominant frequency for the most sensitive-reactive clients.

3. Mapping. Construction of a topographic map of EEG activity, without necessarily providing any feedback, of amplitudes across the 1-30 Hz spectrum across the entire scalp. Electrode site selection in treatment is determined by ranking EEG activity from least to highest in each EEG band, in microvolts amplitude and standard deviation sum for each sensor site. A single channel EEG is used, monitoring each of the standard 10-20 electrode sites in sequence. While amplitude and standard deviation measurements appear to be reliable enough and reasonably correlated with quantitative EEG (QEEG) patterns, measuring correlations among multiple sites is not currently possible since the sites are measured in sequence, and not simultaneously.

4. Treatment providing the feedback in the dose and at the offset frequency as suggested by the above evaluations, in a sequence prescribed by the map.

5. Monitoring the subjective reactions of the patient through self report and the reports of others when available, and the objective changes in the EEG (obtained by periodic remapping) to continue or modify the dosage and site sequences used in the treatment.

6. Involving other tactics to evaluate inferred EEG comodulation (correlated activity in amplitude and/or standard deviation) across the scalp. Comodulation may be responsible for treatment complexity, as well as the duration and stubbornness of their condition.

Most recipients of the LENS input stimulation will have no immediate reaction to the use of this procedure. Some will have relatively short courses of treatment. However, some of those with latent emotional conflicts and intergenerational genetic physiological problems will require longer treatment processes.

Even though this type of stimulation has been found to reduce seizures when they are present, in some patients who have had seizures in the past but where they are not currently present, they have been known to reappear for a brief period of time. Hence the pre-treatment interview is useful in anticipating a complex or problematic treatment. This allows both the therapist and client a chance to review whether the re-experiencing of seizures (or other problems such as anger outbursts, tics, incontinence, or migraines) is something that the client will tolerate.

Reaction Patterns Observed During Treatment. An interesting complexity appears when symptoms become worse during LENS treatment. Many of these patterns we are about to discuss have been considered "side effects." In fact, they may better be considered as stages in treatment that are sometimes experienced in gaining mastery over symptoms. These problems are of five types.

First, vascular type reaction patterns: whether talking about vascular (throbbing pain), periods of anger, rage, sadness, obstinacy, explosiveness, bed wetting (below age six), tics, or convulsions, these episodes become sharper, but shorter in duration, and farther apart in time. As they become increasingly brief, they are experienced increasingly as a fraction of their former intensity, and may not show at all on the surface, in the behavior of the patient. It is often said that as treatment proceeds, the reactions pass faster and have less of a grip on the patient. Finally, their intensity diminishes.

In the end, patients often reflect that circumstances that would have evoked a symptom no longer do. They are completely inarticulate as to what process is happening inside themselves to bring about this change. However, they retrospectively do notice the difference and attribute it to the LENS treatment.

It has been mentioned that the results brought about from the LENS may be either the result of placebo or hypnosis. Yet many of the recipients of the LENS had numerous previous treatments, and many novel ones. Each of these individuals had the opportunity to have hypnosis or placebo work during prior treatment experience. If placebo and hypnosis, either directly or indirectly, have not occurred in the past for these patients, it would seem implausible that the LENS would finally bring them the placebo results that prior attempts had failed to bring. They are involved in receiving the LENS treatment because previous placebos have not worked. Therefore, it is assumed that placebo plays very little part in their current improvement.

Treatment with LENS

It is most important to understand that just starting the use of the LENS does not bring an immediate halt to patient symptoms; in fact, they may appear worse for a while. While these symptoms are ones the patient has had in varying degrees previously and are not caused by the treatment, the change in the way the problem manifests itself and is now experienced is directly attributable to the LENS treatment. The increasing sharpness of these problems, predictable or not, is always of concern for patients, care givers, and referral sources alike. It is also important to know that we expect the therapist to predict and discuss the anticipated changes in how the problems may shift in their manifestations in order to give the patient predictability and confidence in both the treatment process and therapist. A therapist who does not predict this sequence is depriving him or herself of the confidence of the patient. Further, it is important to be considerate of the patient, allowing him or her to choose not to become involved in this approach if the possible consequences are not appealing.

Second, muscular type reactions: muscle contraction pain in non-spastic muscles, and the terrible muscle contraction pain in those with spastic muscles, may occur in head injury, stroke patients, and whenever there is paralysis. Muscle contraction pain of a non-spastic type simply diminishes with time, in contrast to the vascular pattern cited above. There is also pain from the LENS-evoked spasticity reduction that is seen in conditions such as TBI and stroke. This has been in nearly every instance almost intolerable to the patient and those close to the patient. Special care needs to be taken with patients who are hypersensitive to pain medication and are, therefore, unable to use it to alleviate this temporary pain. This intense pain appears to be a function of the decreased bracing offered by non-spastic muscle fibers, which permits the spastic muscles to contract with increasing vigor before they too begin to soften

and relax. When this reaction occurs, the intense pain experienced during spasticity reduction typically lasts from three to five days. It is often accompanied by the sequence of uncontrolled muscle contractions, jumping limbs, increases in sensation, and then the return of partial or complete movements. Note: This kind of pain can be reduced or often completely eliminated with the use of a modality called photonic stimulation.

The third type of reaction is the surprise re-appearance of convulsive or tic-related phenomena that may have long since disappeared. This is actually considered a sub-type of the first class of vascular reactions. These problems re-appear after their long absence, to the near-horror and fright of the parents, care givers, and referral sources. Bed wetting, tics, simple or generalized convulsions, and emotional explosions, may suddenly appear for a few weeks before they subside and make way for higher functioning levels not seen before. Anticonvulsant medication has been extremely useful as an adjunct when the severity of the behavior warrants. The advent of more functional behavior after the cessation of these symptoms has led to the speculation that the untoward behavior had been inhibited by the same mechanisms that kept the patient limited in other ways of functioning. When the behavior has reappeared, and then once again remitted, it may be that the brain found another mechanism to control the aberrant behavior while permitting the flourishing of adaptive and useful skills. Nevertheless, everyone involved needs to provide support, care, and safety in the presence of difficult behavior. To date no one has been caught forever in a trap of regressive, destructive, or bizarre behavior, although the behavior has on rare occasion been extreme and frightening to nearly everybody involved in the very unusual instances when it has occurred.

The fourth type of reaction has been the emergence of adaptive but unvalued, or frankly disvalued, behavior in the patient. Examples of this have been: less fearfulness and greater independence of autistic and Asperger's children, which may be outside of the parents and schools value systems (i.e., children who express anger at siblings when anger is felt to be "bad," children and young adults that become more interested in their own and others' sexuality, children who become more independent, adventurous, and exploratory, and, therefore, begin to take risks which frighten parents; children who voice their own points of view and needs may be contrary to what the parents see appropriate; and children who no longer feel compelled to sit still within the constraints of a rigid school system). All of these behaviors have occurred as greater functioning, greater independence, and greater self-control became more prominent. Some parents who have blanched at the changes in their children will usually keep struggling to be supportive, while other parents have done little but glory at the changes in their children. It is advised to avoid treatment if, in discussions with the patient or family, they are unwilling to risk the occurrence of such behavior. In the approximately two dozen autistic or Pervasive Developmental Disorder children I have treated with the LENS, only one has failed to respond at all, for unknown reasons, while all the rest have delighted their parents with their achievements.

Another example of a positive reaction with untoward effect occurred in the treatment of an older man who had experienced a traumatic brain injury more than a dozen years before he entered treatment. As someone from out of town, he had allocated only a week for treatment before he needed to resume his travels. One of the major problems he had experienced since his head injury was rage, which showed itself in verbal and physical violence. Other problems were chronic angina for which he took medication (and frequent drinks of alcohol from a flask always with him), and a loss of three-dimensional vision. After his first treatment he was freed from heart pain and announced that he no longer needed to drink to control the pain. Within 45 minutes after the treatment he announced that his three-dimensional vision had returned. At first he walked uncertainly as if he was wearing his first pair of trifocals. The next day his wife accompanied him to therapy. He was visibly distressed. She had announced to him that she had suffered his abuse long enough and that she was no longer going to take it–since she no longer had to. She continued to hurl invectives at him and he accused her of trying to destroy the good effects of the treatment. She was offered treatment for the post-traumatic stress which she most certainly

suffered, but she declined. He was asked to be supportive of her in her anger, considering what she lived with for years. Over the next few days under her relentless attacks he regressed to his former state. At the end of treatment they left: him in pain, his three-dimensional vision again lost, and drinking again, and with her as his long-suffering care taker. This illustrates the importance sometimes of working with the entire social system, rather than narrowly focusing on a particular physiological problem in isolation. It also illustrates the inadvisability of working under fixed time limits.

A fifth type of reaction is the recapitulation of previous symptoms, from the most recent to the oldest. Often patients will re-experience first, recent symptoms, and in the last stages of treatment, re-experience symptoms that they experienced as infants. They will often wonder why, for instance, as therapy is about to be completed, they are experiencing abdominal pain. When questioned, they can often remember having such pain or remembering stories of how they had such pain in childhood. These are transient reactions and often pass in a week or so.

Diagnoses. The LENS is a non-specific treatment approach; that is, treatment planning is not guided by diagnosis, which is seen by some as a weakness of LENS treatment. Part of the problem with treating many conditions that have been resistant to amelioration within conventional medical and psychological circles is threefold. First, there is much misdiagnosis. Many of the diagnoses that are proffered are catch basins and euphemisms, and are substitutes for professional ignorance. The problems of diagnoses of many of these conditions, such as Asperger's, Parkinsonian variants, tuberous sclerosis, attention-deficit disorder, fibromyalgia, bipolar disorder, etc., are often beyond the discriminative skills of many practitioners and the most fashionable diagnoses are often used. Second, many conditions are beyond the discriminative capabilities of the diagnostic systems themselves, or their existence as independent entities is controversial and at the whim of what the medical-insurance system will accept given political (turf) and economic considerations. Third, the diagnostic name itself can say little about the treatment when the individual differences among people with the same diagnosis can demand major differences in treatment strategies.

Considerable heterogeneity of brainwave patterns has been found within the broadly defined diagnostic categories. Replacing treatment guided by diagnosis, LENS treatment is predicated on the fact that many psychological and medical conditions involve various types of abnormal EEG activity (Hughes & John, 1999). LENS treatment is designed to reduce abnormal brainwave patterns and is individualized based on the distinctive amplitude and variability patterns found through topographic brain mapping, as well as the patient's subjective reactions to treatment. Finally, it may be said, considering the vast responsibilities of the brain, that the brain, itself, is a non-specific organ. This means that injuries to it may take this shape or that, without any specific predictable outcomes, associated with a particular location, size, depth, or type of injury. Although some outcomes are certain in a gross sense, the particularities of any injury are always some unique combination for the individual involved. The practices of clinicians using the LENS are often filled with almost nothing but patients who are exceptions to medical and psychological predictions of "no recovery possible."

Differences between the LENS and Conventional Photic Stimulation Systems. The LENS differs from currently available consumer (or professional) AVS devices in the following ways. Most of these devices are considered entrainment devices. They lock the brain wave activity on the frequency used to stimulate. The LENS disrupts the way the brain locks onto frequencies, or clusters of frequencies, hopefully helping to free the brain from rigid patterns so that it can have the flexibility to pursue the tasks that it and the person need it to pursue. Second, most of the AVS devices use light frequencies. The LENS uses various frequencies of electromagnetic energy instead of photic stimulation, with is accompanying small risks of evoking a seizure. Light has not been use in most of our applications for the past seven years.

Third, with the LENS, the person's EEG activity controls the frequency of the pulsations in the energy field. This customizes the pulse rate to the person's own activity as it continuously changes. The stimulation frequency of consumer sound and light systems is both pre-programmed and set; a selection is made on the device's front panel, or programmed to change in a way unrelated to the person's actual brain activity. Thus the input stimulation is not individualized to the unique and ever changing brainwave patterns.

Fourth, the LENS uses electromagnetic energy fields infinitesimal in strength, while other devices use much stronger signals. The LENS may, despite the weakness of its energy fields, obtain its power through sustained resonance between the person's EEG activity and the pulsation frequency of the field returned, which may be received by the brain because of its ability to detect patterns. While much of this is speculation, it has been observed that when the resonant pattern of the feedback is broken (when the link between the dominant frequency and the feedback is broken) there are no longer any beneficial effects from our stimulation. That is, when the feedback resonance is broken, both negative as well as positive effects can still appear, but, depending on the frequencies, intensities, and doses involved, they appear with much less consistency and predictability.

A note on the use of the word resonance: Resonance tends to be used in two ways in current medical parlance. In the phrase Magnetic Resonance Imaging, resonance is achieved by the power of the magnetic field on the electrons adding energy to the electrons to move them into higher order shells. Persinger (1974), Sandyk (1994), Rife (1953) and others use the word resonance to refer to a state in which a stimulus intensity or frequency matches a known or theorized fixed frequency in the body. The word "resonance" is used here in a new way in the history of science: that of the changes in the stimulus continuously matching changes in a physical variable (such as brain waves or heart rate). In this sense the resonance is a dynamic one, rather than a static one. Hence, this is a feedback system. However, unlike other biofeedback systems that feed back informational stimuli, the LENS feeds back physical stimuli, the physical properties of which affects physiological changes.

The LENS Equipment Requirements. LENS requires a brain wave measurement device; a computer fitted with an EEG device that controls the emitted energy-field; software to link the brainwaves with the stimulation radio frequency (RF) carrier wave and a system that can deliver levels of energy field feedback at low but precise levels of intensity. These levels are lower in intensity than the electrical field that surrounds digital wrist watches.

In order to provide feedback, the individual is first fitted with the EEG electrodes. In our previous systems, the patient used to wear glasses with components mounted on surface of the lenses, or sat with the glasses mounted on a stand at some distance in front him or her. The operator monitors the computer screen and controls and intensity and duration of feedback so the person remains comfortable. The continued presence of the equipment operator is necessary to watch the quality of the electrode contact, and to determine that the patient preferably remains motionless for a few seconds before the stimulation is given.

While the final determination on how the LENS works must rest with a great deal of research, we believe that the LENS achieves its results by breaking up the rigid, self-protective way the brain has of responding after psychological (stress) or physical trauma and restoring the inhibitory capacity of the cortex.. There is evidence that during any kind of trauma the brain protects itself from seizures and overloads by releasing neurochemicals that protect it from these dangers. Unfortunately, the protection also reduces functional capacity, not unlike the effect of swelling on joint articulation. Long after the trauma is over and the danger is past, the 'protection' may still remain. The person can, therefore, become stuck in various kinds of disabilities due to the reduced neural flexibility of functioning.

Technology Development of the LENS. There was something wrong with nearly all the LENS design elements and procedures from the point of view of those experienced in traditional EEG recording and EEG neurofeedback. This is acutely evident in relation to:

- the established practical concerns regarding shaping reinforcement contingencies
- using visual and/or auditory, or radio frequency feedback carriers for the feedback of information to the brain
- managing high and low frequency EEG activity

- thinking in terms of under- and over-arousal phenomena
- maximizing the amplitudes of some EEG frequencies while inhibiting the amplitudes of other frequencies in relation to particular problems
- locating electrode sites for training
- using topographic maps to provide a treatment plan
- resisting micromanaging the inhibit and reinforcement settings of the EEG in biofeedback treatment
- deferring to subjective reports, rather than quantitative measures of the EEG as either signs of pathology or progress.

There were no clues in the literature for guidance in the preliminary clinical work with the LENS or its predecessors, so the initial treatment guidelines became: Try it on oneself first, always strive to maintain patient's comfort, and cut back if symptoms reflecting over stimulation follow a treatment–even if the post-session discomfort had nothing to do with the treatment.

EEG Site Location. Between 1990 and 1995 the predecessors to the LENS most frequently found success with consistent use of FPZ as the electrode site for the active electrode (with the reference on an ear lobe, and ground at the back of the neck). Depression was typically dispatched in six sessions. This raised the question about the efficacy of choosing any specific site over another at the start of the treatment: one site appeared to be as good as the next when using the precursors to the LENS in the early 1990s. An observation that had no meaning at the time was that delta, primarily, and theta, secondarily, were predominant in the frontal EEG amplitude of nearly all of the patients. In 1995 Ochs wrote a short piece titled *Many Kinds of Depression Are Curable* to spread the good news.

No clear differences in either the way the original light feedback was tolerated or the speed of treatment were found when monitoring the EEG at the sites that were historically popular with traditional EEG biofeedback therapists: occipital locations of O1 and O2, the top of the scalp at CZ, or the site of insult or its contra-coup damage. The central forehead site FPZ was tried because the side effects were minimal, results were as good here as at the other sites, and because it was easier to avoid electrode paste in the hair of the patients during the initial rapport-building session. The frontal site was therefore selected as the point for use at the commencement of treatment. The frontal site has indeed always been more prone to artifact from eye movement, jaw movement, facial expression changes, swallowing, etc. However, since the artifact itself decreased as a function of treatment progression, it seemed plausible to accept the artifact decrease as one of the global indicators of improvement. This suggested the selection of FPZ as an initial starting site. As a consequence, the artifact component of the EEG records was and still is kept, rather than discarded, as is done in conventional neurofeedback treatment.

Another consideration was related to the work of Davidson and Hydahl (1996) and their observation that the left frontal area was less activated in depression. Moving the electrode located at the front-center of the forehead to the left produced, again, no improvement in patients with depressive features. This is not to say that lateralizing the traditional EEG biofeedback might not make a difference in the successful treatment of depression. Using the LENS approach, however, the clinical efficacy of changing the electrode placement to the left frontal area and the practicality of using FPZ overrode all the other considerations pertaining to the selection and use of the more standard electrode sites.

Interestingly, in 1995, with no changes in equipment or software, the selection of FPZ as a site no longer seemed efficacious. In contrast to the delta and theta amplitudes that were predominant in the frontal EEGs of previous patients, alpha now seemed more predominant in the frontal EEGs of those entering treatment. Instead of rapid resolution of depression, irritability and moodiness often resulted from treatment. In contrast to the rapid resolution of depression that had previously been seen, and in contrast to any certainty about how to treat that depression and about placing the active electrode at FPZ, there was no longer any idea about where to place the electrode, either on the basis of the literature or my own experience. This included experimenting with placing the active electrode at C3, C4, OZ, O1, O2, and at CZ. In

an unsystematic way the electrode was moved throughout the standard 10-20 sites. At times there was a remarkable response from sites nobody had talked about; at other times there was no response from any sites addressed.

To better understand what was happening, less expensively than with quantitative EEG brain mapping, single-channel data was collected from all the sites, one site at a time, and this data was fed into Microsoft Excel's surface map. An example of the resulting map is seen in Figure 1, which displays an example of a case with high delta amplitudes throughout the right hemisphere.

A histogram (bar graph) was then created, one bar per electrode site. At first the data made no sense when it was simply organized in the order in which the data was collected. But, when rank-ordered from lowest-to-highest amplitudes for each EEG band, it then appeared that it was a picture of the functionality of the sites– that is, the lower the measured amplitude in microvolts, the more the cortex appeared to be inhibiting the subcortical activity from reaching the cortex so that it could be measured. The greater the inhibitory activity exerted by the cortex, the higher the level of functioning. Figure 2 illustrates the data from Figure 1 in this bar graph format, displaying the amplitudes and standard deviations of the data, rank ordering the electrode sites. The rank ordering became the clue about which sites to select for treatment, and in which sequence. A consistent, organized way to select active electrode sites might be to proceed from those with lowest amplitudes to those with the highest amplitudes. This might not have been the only way to select sites, or necessarily the best way, but at least it was empirical and not based on static experience or research based on aggregated data.

The rationale for this was that in starting with the better-functioning (lower amplitude) sites and proceeding to lower functioning (higher amplitude) sites, the better functioning sites might respond more rapidly and stimulate the more poorly functioning sites. By the time the sites with the lower amplitudes were addressed, the higher amplitudes at other sites would have already decreased, lessening the work that would need to be done. This turned out to be true when the amplitudes were among the highest.

FIGURE 1. LENS Map

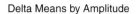

Delta Means by Amplitude

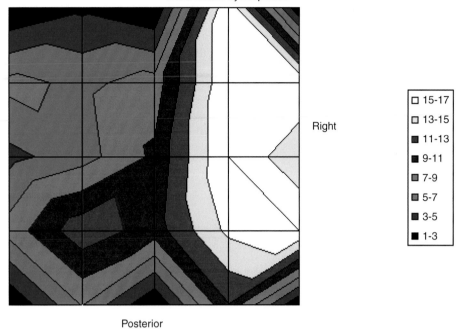

FIGURE 2. Delta Means and Standard Deviations by Sensor Site

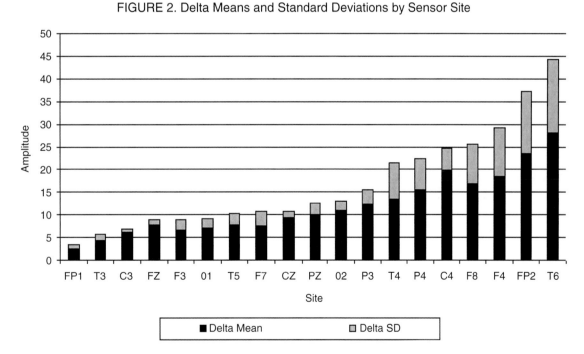

The Need for Mapping. A person's performance can be impaired, even though the EEG activity at any one site is low and smooth across the spectrum. It is necessary to see what kinds of amplitudes are at other sites. It thus became necessary to move away from the forehead site and move the electrode to other sites around the scalp without the historical biases about electrode placement. The next stage was to look at each site for evidences of focal high amplitude and high variability activity, and provide stimulation at that site until the EEG activity was low and stable. The activity at each site was assessed and worked with until ideally no high (> 2.0 μV) amplitude/variability activity was observed.

It also became clear that the information used to make the surface maps could be used to generate treatment plans, specifying the order of sites to be used in treatment. This gives the therapist an empirical basis for starting treatment where the cortex is most functional, and working toward points of less functionality, thereby building upon the patient's strengths in developing their discriminatory capability.

The Beginnings of Mapping. Beginning in 1996, performing inexpensive surface EEG maps that showed the relative amplitude and variability of the EEG at each electrode site (as seen in Figure 1) provided an unexpected treatment benefit, in addition to providing graphic pre and post measures. These maps were acquired by measuring the activity at each site in a specified sequence, using a single-channel EEG instrument. Maps constructed in this way do not allow accurate measurements of the relationships among sites. The unexpected benefit of the sequential maps is that they do provide an explicit plan of which sites to treat, and in what sequence. Beginning at the sites of the lowest activity, and working toward sites with the highest activity, is the same as working from where the cortex is most functional to where it is least functional.

Hyper-Reactivity: Alternating the Polarity of the Leading Frequency (Offset). One of the first clear reactions encountered in the use of precursors to the current LENS was hyper reactivity to the visual feedback stimuli. Initial work began in 1990 with two individuals with post-traumatic stress symptoms (PTSD). Neither had been successfully treated with standard psychotherapy, relaxation training, or with biofeedback (including EEG biofeedback). One of the individuals reacted strongly to the visual and auditory feedback. She jumped in her seat, and complained of a headache and backache.

Later, patients complained about some aspects of the feedback. Some expressed dislike of the "flicker" of the lights. Others complained about the color; others, the brightness. Some could not verbalize the quality they didn't like, but reacted physically, or just said that they didn't like it. Others invoked a variety of verbal and non-verbal startle responses. One individual became explosive and frightened staff members in other rooms with the volume of his outbursts.

In each of these cases, the therapist's response was to change the direction of the leading frequency or offset. If the lights were set to flash at +5 Hz faster than the dominant frequency, the polarity was changed to let them flash at −5 Hz (more slowly than the dominant frequency). In nearly all instances of this problem, changing the polarity of the leading frequency, or offset, decreased the immediate uncomfortable reactions. Further polarity changes at the occurrence of these reactions continued to manage and minimize the reactions. Changing the polarity of the feedback offset was the preferred way to minimize these reactions because the software permitted fast and easy changes of polarity. While a brightness control was available, it involved more time and complex manipulation of the controls.

Alternating polarities had so much impact in the early 1990s that the old procedure, then called EEF (EEG Entrainment Feedback) was modified to allow for specific sequences of pre-programmed polarity alternation. Alternating polarities was one of the important elements of the patent. The alternating polarities seemed to decrease the hyper reactivity of patients. One of the major differences between the approaches in the early 1990s and now is that there are few, if any, immediate reactions of discomfort for which the alternating polarities would be needed. In contrast to the measures taken during those early days, today's strategies tend to be much more subtle.

What's in a Name? The LENS process was originally called EEG Entrainment Feedback (EEF), despite the urging of others, who persisted in the argument that the system seemed to be freeing the brain from being locked up (entraining on itself). The ultimate inspiration for changing the name from EEF to EDF (EEG Disentrainment Feedback) was found in *Chaos: Making of a Science,* by Gleick (1988, p. 293). Gleick used the word "disentrainment," referring to the unlocking of a system. This enabled the precursors to LENS to be seen as disentrainment systems. The name of the process was changed from EEF to EDF. After that, the name changed to Neurophotic Stimulation, to EEG-Driven Stimulation, and finally, to the Flexyx Neurofeedback System (FNS), terms that were less theoretically encumbered and more descriptive names.

It should be emphasized that the treatment effects observed were not due to training to increase some components of the EEG band or inhibit others, even though the observable changes in the EEG activity across the 0 - 40 Hz band appeared comparable to those obtained from the traditional EEG biofeedback training. Experienced EEG clinicians and researchers have been observed attempting to truncate the EEG band activity at one end or the other, or at a selected frequency, either based on some theoretical basis, or previous experience. Early EEF work was also done this way (i.e., attempting to "speed" the EEG by using positive leading frequencies). The system is now run by primarily controlling dosage: the duration of the session and the intensity of the feedback signal.

It is important to understand that in no way, as some people think, is the EEG ever "sped" or "slowed," with the LENS. Under most conditions the amplitude and standard deviation across the spectrum is reduced. Furthermore, this effect is accomplished from the biophysical effects of the feedback signal and its resonance with the EEG of the person, rather than from any reinforcement to elaborate or inhibit the activity in certain bands or frequencies.

Subjects' sensitivity to the brightness of the old visual feedback was recognized while working with Dr. Herbert Gross' patients, a neuropsychiatrist who specialized in head injury. The patients' brightness sensitivity became apparent when the brightness of the lights could not be sufficiently reduced to permit patient comfort. Although good results had been achieved using red LEDs, among the most irritating colors one could employ, the protocol was changed to use green LEDs when it was observed that the red LEDs annoyed the head injured population. This change worked well for the group of head injured patients who had been functioning extremely well prior to their head injuries.

Hypersensitivity. An informal survey of "normal" people, in contrast to those with symptoms, using light stimulation devices available to consumers showed that they enjoyed lights at full brightness. At that time, the operating presumption was the brighter the lights, the better the results. Once the idea was grasped that red lights were both too irritating and too bright, the use of red lights gave way to the more tolerable green ones. The desensitization process was developed gradually, slowly introducing the patients to increased light brightness. This desensitization process allowed them to maintain their comfort with lights of increasing brightness. After desensitizing them to the green lights, it was again possible to use the glasses with the red light-emitting diodes (LEDs), and eventually with continued desensitization, at full brightness in that generation of hardware and software, as well.

While the green LEDs, with their decreased brightness, worked for those who had performed well prior to their head injuries, they were inadequate to meet the sensitivities of a second group of patients with heterogeneous diagnoses prior to their exposure to the LENS, including diagnoses of borderline and various anxiety problems. These patients required green LEDs with tissue paper folded over them, or with masking from manila folder material, and even partial covering from vinyl black electrical tape. Only with such masking could these ultra-hypersensitive patients be comfortable, even with the lights at their lowest intensities. This ultra-hypersensitivity was observed even without light.

As clinical work continued with both head injury and non-head injury patients, it soon became apparent that greater incidence of behavioral and physical pathology seemed to correspond with increasingly prominent hypersensitivity to the visual feedback. In other words, patients with depression, energy problems, irritability, explosiveness, violence, distractibility, short-term memory problems, difficulty in organization, problems following conversation, and difficulty reading, may have all had irritable brains as evidenced by relatively large amplitude, low frequency activity, with relatively high standard deviations. This is an entirely testable hypothesis, and to the extent it is determined to be true, is a rather remarkable statement about human functioning and functional impairment. In fact, diagnosis of hypersensitivity might include much lower level light than is usually used in the detection of photo-hypersensitivity, with more sensitive behavioral observations than frank seizure or EEG spike and wave prominence. This discussion of photohypersensitivity refers to pre-1999 work with the antecedents to current LENS work.

Historical note: The following discussion was applicable when LENS feedback was administered for periods of up to 20 minutes per session. Since 1999, the feedback exposure is typically as brief as one second per electrode site, with an average of four sites worked with during any session, which typically occurs once a week. Thus desensitization pre-1999 was quite different from that which has occurred since then through the present. It is placed here, rather than in an appendix, to give the reader a sense of the flow of the LENS development, as well as to contrast the current practice.

Desensitization. Desensitization used to be a cornerstone of our early work linking EEG with photic stimulation. There is no question that for some patients, desensitization of some type may still be important when they appear to have energy and sudden-onset problems. However, as the mix of patient diagnoses and presenting problems became more complex, and more patients showed fatigue as a major complaint, desensitization began to play a smaller part. At this present time, because the feedback signals, even though not visible, evoke EEG changes much more rapidly than they used to be, it is often not possible to expose patients for a brief enough time to the signals to start the desensitization process. The difference between and one and two seconds can be profound to a very sensitive patient.

With the more recent, briefer treatment durations characteristic of the LENS, there does not seem to be enough time or reason to conduct desensitization the way we used to do it. However, desensitization can still be accomplished through the use of the offset settings. Heredity also plays a part. When parents had a history of mood or energy problems, problems were chronic, or slow in onset, desensitization became less helpful and gave way to the application of feedback with only the gentlest touch, the briefest and least frequent application. For this group, the

therapist using the old I-400 system might use only green lights, masked glasses, and never raise the brightness above "1" in brightness and 1% in duty cycle during the entire course of treatment. Work has been progressing since 1998 using the profoundly low intensity feedback, and while the electromagnetic stimuli are not visible, this still produces changes in the EEG when the EEG is observed after the feedback stimulus has been given.

Here is an example of how the need for desensitization was discovered in the original systems. Ordinarily, the brightness of the lights was varied frequently during a treatment session and over the course of treatment. Just discussing the brightness of the lights, and none of the other treatment variables such as electrode site, for example, an intensity of "1" may have been used during the first six sessions. As the sessions progressed, symptom intensity decreased. In the seventh through the tenth session, intensity was increased to a brightness of "2." In the eleventh through the thirteenth sessions the brightness was increased to "4." In other words, not only was the brightness increasing, but the pace of increase was coming more and more rapidly as time progressed. Perhaps in the fourteenth session the brightness was increased three times, from "6" to "18" to "36." The brightness ratings are in quotation marks because they are arbitrary in value. No luminosity values were ever formally evaluated for the numerals used to indicate brightness. Yet the brightness values were linearly controlled by current flow; so that relative to each number, a brightness of "2" is half that of "4." Whereas initially going from "1" to "2" would have been uncomfortable for this hypothetical patient, in the end leaping from "18" to "36" would have been quite comfortable. In the meantime, symptom intensities across the entire range would commonly have dropped precipitously.

During one session, by accidentally using new software with a hidden defect, a protocol was loaded that held the light frequency low and constant during the feedback periods, revealing EEG activity which was initially seen when the patient's complaints were prominent. A young woman in her thirties, otherwise high functioning, complained of a post-puberty history of premenstrual fatigue, irritability, racing thoughts and sleeping problems, leaving her with severely restricted professional job functioning fifty per cent of the time each month. She left her job to avoid the continuous, extreme effort needed to fulfill her professional duties two weeks of each month. For two menstrual cycles after desensitization had been completed, her sleep problems ceased, as did her racing thoughts, irritability, and diurnal fatigue. During her third premenstrual cycle, however, her fatigue returned and was ever present. Examination of her EEG spectrum recorded under moderately bright light showed relatively large amounts of high amplitude, low frequency activity when the brightness was consistent across all four feedback periods. The session was constructed using a one-minute, no-feedback pre-baseline, four 18-second periods of feedback (during which feedback stimulation may or may not be given), and a one-minute no-feedback post-baseline, all repeated 17 times. All recording was done eyes closed. The electrode site was Cz, with a left-ear reference.

The high amplitude, low frequency activity was not present when the light brightness was reduced to 10% during the first and third 18-second feedback-possible periods. The informal hypothesis that alternating brightness would have no effect in accelerating change in EEG amplitudes seemed patently wrong. Alternating flashes between the left and right eye succeeded in lowering the amplitude of the EEG more than when we lowered the brightness of the feedback light stimulation, perhaps because there was only half as much stimulation being given.

At the current time, the intensity of the feedback signals (which are no longer photic stimulation) are so weak, their effects so strong, and the treatment times necessarily so short, that issues of desensitization have taken a back seat to dosage. The exposures are now so short that it has been difficult to see how to manage a desensitization program. It has not been until recently that six years of experience with the low power electromagnetic carrier wave feedback has allowed us to understand how to begin to integrate our prior experience with lights into current LENS work. Currently, increasing the number of electrode sites that we work with during each session, decreasing the interval between sessions, and decreasing the offset frequency at which we provide the stimulation are all ways to increase the power of the feedback stimulation and treatment dose.

Desensitization and Level of Functioning. Another past observation, equally testable, was that the level of some patients' functioning consistently increased as their comfort increased with progressively brighter light feedback. This means that depression, irritability, reactions to bright or interrupted light, impatience and explosiveness lifted, non-focal pain decreased, violence ceased, distractibility, anxiety reactions, organization, problems following conversation, and difficulty reading were all markedly ameliorated–without any claim that they were totally erased. The problems were improved enough that friends, spouses, distant relatives, employers, and last, the patients, themselves, were delighted and surprised at the improvement. Academic grade improvements were noticed as well. These observations were echoed by physicians and neuroscientists not involved in this treatment (although no attempt was made to keep them blind to who was involved in the treatment). In retrospect, it may have been that the enhanced ability of the cortex to inhibit electrophysiological reactions from the increased brightness of the feedback stimulation was the sign that the cortex had repaired itself. In contrast, if someone's brain had become re-traumatized, it was very difficult to re-desensitize the person for unknown reasons.

We learned that it was not always possible to desensitize someone. Desensitization was indicated especially when a person was energetic, and less useful when the person often felt fatigued. It is also possible that new techniques will permit successful partial desensitization of those people otherwise unable to tolerate the standard process.

Pace of Desensitization. There was a characteristic desensitization curve, even though the entire desensitization process could take anywhere from five minutes to five months. The initial pace of desensitization was always relatively slow, relative to its much higher rate of change at the end of the treatment process. The desensitization curve appeared to have been an accelerating curvilinear function in which the slope of the rate of change of the light intensity was often imperceptible initially, but its rate of change was geometric at the end. Put another way, the initial brightness changes may be 1% at a time, but increase in units to 20% at a clip occurred in the final minutes of the process.

We found that during a long desensitization process, lasting months, the final 80% of the brightness changes may occur in one treatment session. This pattern was consistent across all patients whenever the need for desensitization was present. The desensitization curve was reminiscent of the logarithmic curves in the Weber-Fechner law of perception, in which brightness increases logarithmically with the absolute value of the brightness of the stimulus. The observation of the adaptation of the brain may cast light on the flip side of the brightness estimation: that is, on the place that the rate of reconnectivity of the cortex plays as it regains competence.

Decreasing Light Intensity After Desensitization. One patient, early in the exploration of the LENS, suffered workplace abuse trauma and re-experienced symptoms formerly minimized by the LENS. She remained free from her former dislike of the brighter lights, however. There was the implication that she had not relapsed into photosensitivity and, therefore, did not need a lowering of the light intensity. Continued treatment with the LENS at high levels of intensity, however, did not lead to a decrease in her new trauma symptoms, which showed themselves prominently as depression, anxiety, and anger. High amplitude and variability in low EEG frequency bands again showed itself in her record. It was hypothesized that the intensity might be re-stimulating her pathology (i.e., perpetuating her re-traumatization). As a test of this hypothesis the intensity of the lights was drastically lowered and almost immediately she reported a decrease in her depression. During this same period, Russell was using the LENS with a few patients who had experienced cerebral vascular accidents. He applied this change in approach to the therapy he was doing and found that motoric and cognitive rehabilitation progress was stimulated and accelerated by lowering the intensity of the lights.

Interestingly, many users of pre-programmed frequency, commercially-available sound and light systems run their systems at full intensity. The colors and patterns are visually interesting at full intensity. The patients most often will seek full intensity, partly for aesthetic reasons, and partly, upon questioning, because they think that brighter is inherently better and that all treatments inherently involve the struggle to tolerate discomfort–which they feel they should do if they really want to improve.

However, it is probably not legitimate to equate the stimulation from fixed or ramping frequencies of the audio-visual stimulation (AVS) systems with that of the LENS and its predecessors. The AVS systems' stimulation intensity may be seen as ambient light, or "noise" stimulation, not nearly so tightly related to the living, dynamic EEG. This may be supported by the observation that AVS users need to use much brighter light intensities than what was ever used in the LENS predecessors. It seems to me that the inherent resonance of the LENS-type stimulation allows the LENS stimulation to remain at very low intensity and still have dramatic physiological and behavioral effects. It is apparently not the case that brighter is always better, nor that tolerating increased discomfort will accelerate recovery. In fact, when comfort is used as a cue for intensity settings, and the feedback LENS intensity is minimized, improvements in energy, mood, and cognitive integrity are often noted. This has been our experience with our older light stimulation system and with the newer versions of LENS.

When the LENS treatment is completed, the cortex may be in a very different state than it was at the start of treatment. Whether or not patients had been desensitized, the patients were, in fact, more receptive to and discriminating about external stimuli, but not hypersensitive or hyper-reactive. Their responses were more flexible and appropriate to the level of feedback present in the moment. In view of the greater sensitivity, is it any wonder, then, that high intensity, strobic feedback would act as if it was overloading the cortex of these individuals and in a sense replicating the internally-produced pathology that once was there? Decreasing the feedback stimulation after the desensitization process might be more effective because the brain has, through the course of treatment, become more responsive to feedback.

The pathology of some brains may require a major change or reorganization at the start of therapy, and trying to work locally at the site of damage may not be useful if the person is very energetic. Once the brain has been globally re-organized by the desensitization process and the patient is comfortable at full intensity, continued feedback at the peak level of intensity may now overwhelm the cortex. This represents a method by which one may safely experiment with replicating trauma and recovery from trauma. After desensitization, by lowering the intensity of the feedback, we may be more able to locally stimulate the cortex–something that we were unable to do at the start of treatment. At this stage in treatment, behavioral changes may be more closely tied to what is commonly thought of as local cortical neuro-psychological functions. In other words, local site feedback and local site recovery may be addressable only after global feedback and reorganization has taken place. This might also mean that following LENS treatment, further localized treatment with traditional neurofeedback might have more affect than it would have had previously.

In an interesting side note, a highly functional scientist was put on an older LENS system, and not only felt nothing, but was unable to be overdosed by extremely high levels of brightness. It may be that one of the defining aspects of functioning well is that the brain is able to flexibly respond to high stimulation input, at least in relatively short exposures.

Cortical Permeability. In the early days of using EEG-driven feedback, it was noticed that the EEGs of high-functioning individuals were rather quiet, low amplitude recordings. In contrast, the EEGs of dysfunctional and physically traumatized individuals were typically filled with high-amplitude, low frequency band activity. Recollect that the cortex is one of the last organs to develop both ontogenetically and phylogenetically. The ostensive purpose of the cortex is to provide the integration and inhibition of subcortical brain center activity, which results in the appearance of our higher functioning capabilities.

The appearance of this EEG slowing that is seen as high amplitude delta, theta, and alpha activity, has been, in the view of traditional EEG and neurofeedback circles, considered a problem. Activity in these frequency bands is often inhibited during neurofeedback. Discussion of delta, theta, and alpha excesses was and is often prominent in exchanges of ideas about

treatment. Yet delta, theta, and alpha activity may not be the entire problem because activity in these bands is commonly present when higher functions are not engaged.

Occasional high amplitude activity in low frequencies (which is often seen as pathological) may be present in individuals who not only function well, but who are exceptionally creative. These exceptions are not understood. Thus one needs to be careful about glibly pathologizing all EEG slowing, just as spinal anomalies were overly pathologized early in the history of MRI.[1]

In individuals having problems, however, the presence of activity in these slower frequency bands may translate into sections of the cortex, by their impaired inhibitory functioning, permit the delta, theta, and alpha activity to show themselves and be recorded at the scalp. That is, these areas of the cortex no longer function properly, and do not inhibit the low frequency activity. It is the poor functioning of the cortex that fails to inhibit the physiology that gives rise to the excessive EEG activity, which allows the high amplitude EEG activity to be recorded; that is the problem–not the activity itself. The task, then, of the treatment is to bring back the functioning of these impaired sections of the cortex. The sign that these areas are returning to normal function is twofold. First, the EEG amplitudes become inhibited and lower. Second, functional improvement results. The object is to reduce the permeability of the cortex so that it regains its inhibitory and integrative functions. This, in turn, permits higher functioning to return.

Decreases in the Amplitude and Variability of Low Frequency Activity. There were, and are, decreases in EEG amplitude and variability that accompany LENS feedback if the initial amplitudes are high enough. Decreases appear across the entire 1-30 Hz spectrum, but especially in the low frequency 1-12 Hz EEG range, including that activity which is clearly and even probably attributable to artifact.

These decreases are sensitive to the level of intensity of the feedback. There is a window at any time in which the feedback intensity will decrease the amplitude and variability. If the intensity is too low or too high–a Yerkes-Dodgson curve–amplitude reduction will not occur. In fact, if the intensity is (resonant and) too high, the amplitudes may rise, as mentioned above.

The range of intensity in which the amplitudes drop will vary with the phase of treatment. For those with the energy and stamina, higher levels of feedback will decrease amplitudes and standard deviations early in the treatment. As treatment progresses and the patient becomes more sensitive and less hyper reactive, the intensity will need to be reduced in order to continue to reduce the levels of activity. Reducing the level of intensity is necessary to reduce the amplitude and standard deviation, and to increase the functioning the patients.

These evoked (by feedback) amplitude and variability reductions may reflect, on a neuronal level, organic events which parallel the recovery of energy, mood, and cognitive capacities. These alterations in functional reactivity appear to represent the quieting of the brain, and the containing of emotional and attentional impulses in a state of ambient readiness. The recovery of skill was apparent in both those who had clear mechanical and physical trauma, and those who suffered lifelong energy, emotional, anxiety, and cognitive functional problems.

This lowering of the EEG's amplitude using the LENS stands in contrast to other attempts to increase amplitudes of the same EEG bands using traditional EEG biofeedback. Whether it is the feedback itself, the desensitization process, alternate offset polarity, or some other element of the procedure that automatically affects the amplitude and variability decrease, the key point is that these decreases occur in the LENS process without the treatment directing this, which is so characteristic of traditional EEG biofeedback. The implication is that some element(s) in the LENS treatment process triggers a self-organizing/corrective mechanism in the brain which optimizes functioning, and which requires no conscious involvement of the individual receiving the feedback.

In addition to the frequent appearances of EEG slowing, we encounter infrequent instances of patients with EEG suppression, or very low amplitude and low standard deviation EEG activity. These have been most frequently seen in chronic fatigue and fibromyalgia, and usually interlaced with depression. Depression, seen apart from occurrences of chronic fatigue, is most often accompanied by elevation in EEG activity. Ordinarily we have screened out those with unusually low amplitude EEG activity (less than 1 µV) because they have been particularly refractory to our methods.[2]

One more type of EEG activity is important to mention: normal or high amplitude EEG activity, accompanied by standard deviations of below 1. The EEGs of those with these abnormally smooth EEG recordings are often seen to show dramatic rises in elevation following LENS treatment, often accompanied by increases in functioning. This appears to be a due to a treatment-induced lifting of suppression of the EEG. The increase in functioning may be due to the freeing of energy bound by the neurochemistry of suppression. Those with problems functioning speak of the enormous effort it takes to think, organize, plan–in short to compensate for both their symptoms and due to the suppressive effects of neurochemical protection.

Diagnostic Considerations. The LENS has been successfully and reliably used with autism, Asperger's syndrome, post-concussive disorders, depressive disorders, post-traumatic stress disorders, attention deficit disorder with and without hyperactivity, chronic fatigue syndrome, fibromyalgia, and spastic paresis following cerebral vascular accidents. The improvements have been significant enough to have made noticeable differences in the lives of patients, both at home and at work. It may be more useful to think about the above disorders as variations of a single disorder (cortical permeability or insufficiency), in which the cortex is inadequate to the task of inhibiting the bioelectrical activity.

The Potential Central Locus of "Peripheral" Problems. Most pathology is treated peripherally, even when there are known central nervous system mechanisms. To date, peripheral treatment has been attempted though exercise, diet, etc., except where frank neuroleptic or neurosurgical intervention has been involved. For instance, fibromyalgia is typically seen as a muscle problem, since the tender points have been muscular, even though the balance problems, mental fog, and fatigue are typically seen as central problems.

The LENS provides a behavioral way to directly influence central mechanisms versus the indirect means used in traditional EEG feedback. With the LENS, the signals picked up from the brain are ultimately fed back into the tissues of the brain. The information the LENS feeds back to the brain has no graphic or symbolic meaning, as does the information from traditional EEG neurofeedback, so there is nothing to interpret. However, while the information is fed back directly into the brain, it is also not targeted (i.e., certain frequencies are not associated with particular functions) and there is no selectivity of where the feedback signals go in the brain.

It is true, however, that only one site at any one time establishes the resonance source for the feedback and that is the site of the active electrode. So while the feedback is believed to permeate all of the brain tissues and is non-specific in that sense, it remains resonant only with the site of the active electrode, the site whose dominant frequency is generating the basis for the feedback signal (feedback frequency = dominant frequency + offset).

The extent of the promise of this approach can only be imagined. Emerging theories of brain function, specifically with regard to the self-organizing capability of the brain, will find the LENS a significant intervention model for both clinical treatment and pathology simulation studies.

The Corrected Technical Inadequacy Uncorrected: Alternating Hemispheric Feedback. One of the more interesting sides of exploring the LENS has been the extent to which preconceptions about accuracy have been unnecessarily attached to efficacy. There were clear inaccuracy problems in our first generation software, causing the left and right lights to strobe 180 degrees out of phase. It was assumed that they had been flashing in phase synchrony. When the lights flashed at lower frequencies, however, they were observed to flash together only inconsistently. The asynchronously flashing lights were called to the attention of the programmer with the intention of emphasizing how remarkable it was to obtain good results with phase dyssynchrony.

As the second generation software was developed, left-right flash phase synchrony was initially looked at as an imprecise sloppiness, and not included. While the desensitization process seemed identical in the second-generation system, the results seemed to hold less

well–until the programmer was persuaded to supply an option for permitting the lights to strobe 180 degrees out of phase. Additionally, it was suggested that alternating hemispheres were stimulated with the left-right alternating feedback. This strategy seemed to inhibit high voltage activity relatively rapidly across the spectrum. The use of alternating light feedback was especially useful later in treatment. Using alternating feedback as the first element of treatment prevented treatment from having the carry-over between sessions that it did when it was used later in treatment, wherein it appears to amplify treatment effects. The transfer of learning value from alteration of phase later in treatment may correspond developmentally with the acquisition of stereoptic vision.

Initially, it looked as if the work with alternating sides flashing might be an example, subject to experimental verification, of the power of accidental digressions from pre-planned designs. Initially it looked as if the left-right alternating stimulation was extremely significant in a number of ways. However, years later, the question changed as to whether this was just another way of reducing the intensity of stimulation, only providing 50% of the intensity at any one time. This question could be resolvable now by doing a thorough analysis of the electromagnetic field emitted by any visual stimulation device so that the concurrent visual and electromagnetic influences can be understood for their individual contribution to any observed phenomena.

Consciousness Is Optional. Psychologists and traditional biofeedback therapists tend to hold to the model of treatment as a conscious process. Yet an unknown percent of patients receive therapy that is primarily conversational for long periods of time with minimal concrete results (even though they may report feeling better). Non-psychotherapeutic psychiatrists, on the other hand, tend to see medication as the primary component in the recovery and symptom alleviation/management process, relegating the patient's conscious participation and learning a secondary, if not functionally irrelevant role.

The LENS appears to offer a behavioral non-pharmacologic, non-surgical and non-psychotherapeutic way to influence behavior, cognitive function, and feeling states, especially with regard to symptoms that result from mechanical and/or psychological trauma. LENS is behavioral and not medical because the signals are profoundly minimal in intensity. It seems likely that functioning, and not structure is directly influenced; the adaptability of the individual and subsystems of the individual are influenced, and adaptability is learning.

Our subjects show significant decreases in EEG amplitude and standard deviation without specific instructions to suppress this activity. LENS, therefore, complements both pharmacologic and psychotherapeutic techniques. Conscious self-development associated with psychotherapy can be valuable, but can proceed better when the patient's consciousness is clearer and thereby more able to process information.

Is It Self-Regulation Even Though It Is Not a Conscious, Deliberate Process? The use of the LENS has been criticized as inducing passive change in the patient, which has little chance of promoting either a sense of empowerment or long-term change in the patient's psychological status. It is here hypothesized that the LENS, instead, shortens treatment by eliminating a major portion of the time-consuming feedback process, clarifies the patient's tendencies to control the inner flow of conscious experience, and still permits the chance to desensitize, drop defenses, and allow neurochemistry to return to productive homeostasis. Further, the EEG disentrainment supports, but does not force, the patient to experience unfamiliar states of consciousness that enhance the chances of recognizing these states with further treatment. While the person receiving the LENS treatment may feel as if they are "not doing anything" and are not involved in a conscious learning process, they have nonetheless brought themselves to a setting that is structured to allow their brain to adapt and learn at a neurological level.

Traditional neurofeedback therapy undoubtedly contributes to the acquisition of self-regulatory skills, as well as operantly conditioning healthier brainwave patterns. However, the elimination of the lengthy and hard work in front of a computer screen with LENS treatment still seems to promote acute patient awareness of the operation of his or her defensive structure and process. The acquisition of a state of passive-allowing of experience seems facilitated by the LENS as it increases the patient's awareness of being drawn into different states of consciousness.

Most of our self-regulatory processes are non conscious, and not voluntary. To take on a mission of micromanaging even a significant portion of these non conscious processes seems to me to significantly reduce one's available conscious resources for tasks usually requiring large amounts of consciousness: learning new skills, and appreciating and enjoying life. It seems ideal to me to find ways to maximize our non conscious skills, so that we can find greater ease and clarity for our conscious lives.

Is the EEG Really Necessary to Drive the Feedback? This question is of central importance. If the EEG is unnecessary to enhance the clarity and ease of our conscious experience, then ways can be found much less expensively to efficaciously use the fixed and/or pre-set frequency feedback in treatment.

There were several inadvertent triple blind studies conducted during the history of the LENS. Triple blind studies are ones where even an experimenter does not know who gets what procedures. Not only were the subjects and machine operators blind to the study, but I knew only in retrospect exactly what happened. Unbeknownst to me or anybody else, during the use of our earlier light feedback system, it was discovered that the EEG had somehow been disconnected from the lights and that the flash rate had remained at 4 Hz regardless of the instrument readings to the contrary. After some investigation it became clear that there was a bug in the program, installed by accident by the programmer after he "upgraded" the software. This bug prevented any change in the LENS programming without effectively disconnecting it from the EEG.

Reviewing the records of the half-dozen patients seen during the time of the problem, all were found to have regressed during the period that the EEG was disconnected from the visual feedback. They were all either more hypersensitive, or more depressed. Patients were provided with enough free treatment to correct the problem and they began to progress again.

This experience yielded several different conclusions. First, it appears that using the EEG to influence the feedback stimulation rate is indeed necessary and useful. Second, programs that were developed that intuitively compensated for the irritating fixed-frequency feedback by dropping the intensity of the light feedback that was originally used further reinforced the utility of very low intensity levels. Third, the default fixed frequency was changed from 4 Hz to 20 Hz, to guard against inadvertent delta and theta feedback occurring in the event of a programming error. Last, considering the actual effects of over stimulation conditions in replicating pathological states and functioning, it may be possible that we can better study central nervous system problems by using the proper kinds and levels of feedback stimulation to experimentally replicate and even temporarily evoke problems in the brain to more accurately study brain functioning, impairment and recovery.

Frequency of Treatments. The optimal treatment schedule is one that leaves the individual refreshed. There is no treatment schedule that affects everybody the same way. Treatments can be effective when delivered on a daily basis if the patient can tolerate this level of feedback. On the other hand, it is possible to leave the patient slightly disoriented, fatigued, and with a headache from sessions which are too frequent or long in duration, or where the offset is too low. While each patient is different, these factors generally underlie clients' reported post-session discomfort. With such patients, much less frequent treatments may be the ones that speed the course of treatment the most. Treatment effects do appear to need a critical mass of treatments to overcome the rigidity of the system that perpetuates the symptom systems and pathology.

The therapist must be willing to rely on the signs of subjective discomfort of the patient, such as fatigue, rigidity, obsessiveness, and depression that will not respond, and be willing to take the risk of giving too little feedback by reducing the stimulation even to such small amounts that it seems ridiculous (i.e., one second per month) if need be. Thus while the range of feedback intensity dose can be enormous (e.g., ranging from three sessions/day to six seconds per week) the primary cues for decision making all come from the patient to the therapist who is willing to risk anxiety and the appearance of being foolish, but who will, to advance the welfare of the patient, reduce feedback intensity.

One of the seductive elements in the use of the LENS is that longer treatment sessions can appear to work well for some treatment populations, such as autistic children. This may fit into preconceived ideas that a therapist may have about the necessity of lengthier sessions. The consequence of longer sessions is that while they work in the short term, on a week-to-week basis they contribute to a slower pace for the occurrence of improvements. The therapists maintain that longer sessions do work for this population. My response is "But have you tried briefer . . . ?"

Duration of Treatment and Factors that Determine Treatment Length. The degree of sensitivity to the LENS feedback, how rapid the rate of desensitization, and the pre-existing duration of the symptoms and efforts to compensate for them are the best determinants of the duration of treatment. For example, the average duration of treatment for a formerly high functioning, multi-tasking patient who had a head injury 2.5 years prior to treatment, is approximately 6 sessions with seven or fewer seconds of feedback during each session. If the person had lifelong problems prior to the trauma, the treatment time ranges from 40 to 70 sessions. If the problem is severe post-stroke or spinal cord bruising paresis, the course of treatment may number into the hundreds of sessions. However, for those with mild to moderate stroke, even with paralysis, shocking relief from paralysis may be seen in between 6 and 14 sessions. An average of three sessions has produced startling results with people who have been overly stressed by work and/or home conditions over several years. No matter if the patient is suicidal, if they were high functioning before the protracted stress their treatment has averaged three sessions.

Reducing Treatment Time with Offsets. The antecedent systems to the LENS were designed with offsets from the start, originally to reduce the chance of elaborating a seizure that might have been triggered by the original bright flashing feedback lights. At that time offsets were called "leading frequencies," because it was thought that they led the dominant frequency to rise or lower. The term "offset" was felt to be more descriptive.

If the feedback signal frequency could never equal the peak, or dominant frequency, two effects were anticipated. First, the feedback frequency might not elaborate seizure activity if there was a tendency toward seizing. Second, the offset feedback frequency might shift energy away from the seizure frequency, which would be the peak EEG frequency at that time. In drawing energy away from the dominant frequency, the amplitude of the dominant frequency would be lowered, corresponding to the effect ordinarily seen.

Defining Frequency Offset. The offset evaluation originated from examining patient data in a typical year-end review. Up to that time we rotated through each of the standard offsets of 5, 10, 15, and 20 Hz at each site we treated. During one particular year-end review of data it was noticed that patients considered more sensitive showed lower EEG amplitudes during the periods when higher offsets (15 or 20 Hz) were used; and patients considered more reactive and less sensitive showed lower EEG amplitudes during the periods when the lower offsets (5 or 10 Hz) were used. If higher functioning levels accompanied lower amplitudes, then it might be wasting time to expose patients to offsets that didn't do much to lower their amplitudes. The task then became to design an evaluation that demonstrated the EEG response to each of the standard offsets. It initially used a baseline of one minute, followed by each of the offsets, structured as follows:

- One second of feedback with an offset of 5, followed by one minute of post baseline monitoring
- One second of feedback with an offset of 10, followed by one minute of post baseline monitoring
- One second of feedback with an offset of 15, followed by one minute of post baseline monitoring
- One second of feedback with an offset of 20, followed by one minute of post baseline monitoring

To reduce the possibility that relaxing during the 1-minute baseline would affect the EEG amplitudes during the stimulation, the baseline was lengthened to six minutes to be sure that the patient had stabilized in relaxation before being

exposed to the first offset. If the amplitudes of delta and alpha are measured after exposure to feedback at different offsets from the measure dominant frequency, the amplitudes resulting from each offset can be assessed. The offset that produced the lowest band amplitude would be the one to select during treatment to achieve maximum decrease in amplitude activity.

The problem with providing several different offsets in an evaluation, if the offsets are presented in the same order, time after time, is that order effects may be influencing the results. In fact, it is probably true that order effects influence the observed responses of EEG amplitudes to the offsets. To randomize the order of presentation, however, brings its own problems. In order to prevent the patient from being over stimulated, there is limited opportunity to present stimulation during any one session. Offset evaluations ordinarily provide a significant dose of four seconds of stimulation, and are reserved for those patients who are sturdy enough to tolerate them. So it seems inadvisable to do a comprehensive presentation of stimulation with counterbalanced orders of presentation and hope to find the "real" or "right" offset. Rather, the offset evaluation is viewed as a starting place from which to derive the offset.

Interestingly, it was found that the numbers defined as offsets have face validity. A patient who is reasonably insensitive and foggy at the start of the treatment will often have an offset closer to 5 or 10 Hz. If the patient, in later treatment, declares that they are not much clearer and better functioning, one would expect that a repeat offset evaluation will show the offset redefined at a higher number. The patient, then, will also seem more discriminant, less foggy, and more functional. And in fact, the repeat offset evaluation often redefines the offset at closer to 20.

Figure 3 displays an example of an offset evaluation. It shows the response of the delta frequency band amplitude and standard deviation to one second of feedback stimulation at the four different offset frequencies of 5, 10, 15, and 20 Hz. It can be seen that the most effective offset frequency for reducing delta was 5 Hz.

Does the EEG Change with LENS Stimulation? There is usually a question in the minds of both the prospective patient as well as the pro-

FIGURE 3. Delta Response to Different Offsets

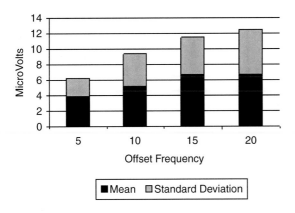

spective therapist about whether the LENS actually changes the EEG. After all, therapists using traditional neurofeedback complained that they saw relatively little change in the EEGs of some of their patients. While change in the EEG itself may or may not be correlated with achieving the kind of change that a patient wants, at least it can serve as encouragement that something positive may happen sooner rather than later. The offset evaluation has three purposes. First, as above, it empirically defines an offset. Second, it provides a chance for the non-sensitive patient to put a toe in the water and experience a standardized dose of feedback. If the patient is known to be very reactive (e.g., to light, sound, medications, weather changes, foods, odors, and other people), one can presume an offset of 20, and use a less demanding procedure than the offset evaluation to provide an experience. In either case we use a test dose of feedback stimulation to be as sure as we can that the experience leaves the patient comfortable. Finally, we can compare the baseline and feedback sections of the evaluation to see if the EEG has changed in amplitude and standard deviation.

We have two choices in selecting an offset frequency to use in LENS sessions. One choice is to use the graph of delta responses to the alternative offset frequencies. The other choice is to use the alpha responses. Delta activity has always seemed more responsive than alpha activity, perhaps because alpha activity may be more genetically determined. Therefore, we use the graph of delta activity for selecting our offset frequency. This choice has proven more suc-

cessful than using alpha offset for reducing elevated amplitudes across the frequency spectrum. In addition, delta offset responses are favored over the reactions to offsets within the theta band because clinical experience has shown that using delta offset data was most effective in reducing both delta and theta activity (in comparison with using theta offsets).

In Figure 4 it is clear that delta amplitude and standard deviation dropped from the baseline following feedback. In contrast to Figure 3, this figure presents the average of data from all four of the offsets. However, it also shows that alpha amplitude and standard deviation slightly increased. This demonstrates that measurable EEG changes can be documented in a brief ten minute evaluation, with as little as four seconds of feedback being given during that time.

Reducing Treatment Time with Brain Mapping. Quantitative EEG (QEEG) was discontinued in the early 1990s because it did not offer clear and reliable guidance in defining which sites to work with and in what sequence. The LENS practitioners were seeking treatment planning answers about patients who presented more complex problems. These problems created uncertainty about how best to bring about progress, and especially in choosing electrode sites. A useful mapping system would graphically specify the order and sequence of sites to treat. The operational definition of an "appropriate" electrode site is one with reduced evoked EEG amplitude within five minutes.

It has been our clinical experience that by simply mapping the amplitude and standard deviation of the EEG at 19 or more electrode sites, we can specify electrode site sequencing and placement. As a basis for treatment planning with LENS this seems to speed the rate of EEG change, wasted treatment time is avoided, and discomfort is minimized by choosing and treating multiple electrode sites during each session, following an order from lowest amplitude/variability to greatest amplitude/variability.

EEG Coherence Issues. EEG coherence is correlated phase activity in a frequency band between different EEG sites. Variability in the form of standard deviations can also be correlated, but is usually not talked about in relation to coherence across electrode sites. Interestingly a major EEG reference makes no mention of coherence in its index (Niedermeyer & da

FIGURE 4. Offset Evaluation: Averaged Frequency and Standard Deviation Changes

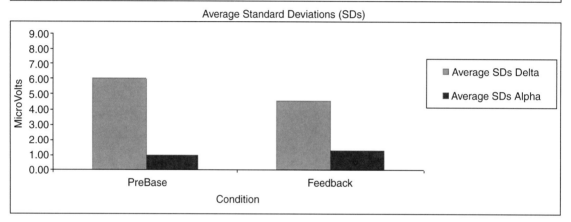

Silva, 1999) making the following discussion highly speculative.

The Clinical Side of Coherence. There are patients who are easier to treat, and those who are more complex. "Easier" means that amplitudes reduce and stay low at the sites treated. The easier patients do not suffer an exacerbation of their symptoms after initial treatments. "Complex" means that (a) frequency band amplitude at any site may increase after it lowers, (b) another frequency band may increase in activity at the site monitored, (c) band amplitudes at the same site may see-saw (alpha and delta amplitudes may see-saw), (d) band amplitudes at one site may fall while the same band amplitudes may rise at a different site, and (e) symptoms may flare up after the session. Coherence problems may be recognized by any of these items. On the topographic maps, map areas showing pools of the same color are, in fact, showing areas with the same amplitudes of activity within a frequency band. The sites, then, have correlated amplitudes which may reflect the probability of high coherence. A review of 100 topographic maps, sorted into piles of low-to-high areas of similar amplitude was roughly correlated with patients who were, respectively easy-to-hard to treat. This evaluation was crude and bears systematic and precise investigation.

Hunches About Coherence and Systems. Correlated activity may mean that the activity occurs in a system, an integrated pattern. As with any system, the activity as a whole behaves different than the behavior as the sum of the parts. Changes in the activity at specific sites that are part of a system would be expected to be more resistant to change, and especially to lasting change. Therefore, it is expected that a system would need to be worked with as a whole system, rather than at just at one or two sites.

Components of Systems. There are three major components of systems: (a) sites that are not involved in a system, (b) sites that react to the activity in a system and either amplify the systems activity or dampen the system's activity, and (c) the generators of the system's activity, influenced by the other components. When a site responds to treatment and remains affected without rebounding after the session, it acts as if it is unrelated to the system. If there were no system present, as is sometimes the case, the person would experience a "miracle," a sudden and noticeable reduction in symptoms.

Ramifications of Coherence for the LENS Treatment Planning: A Story. As a metaphor, let's say that there are three types of people in a riotous intersection. First, there are the bystanders. They are the ones who are easily moved by those trying to reduce the noise in the intersection. They are not particularly involved in the activity, and do not contribute to the noise. But their presence does encourage the others fomenting the noise.

Second, there are the collaborators. They have varying degrees of interest and involvement in generating the noise in the intersection. They provide reinforcement and energy for the instigators of the noise and they derive satisfaction from their involvement. The degree of ease with which the collaborators can be moved is a function of their relationship with the instigators, and with the amount of energy they have. Last, there are the instigators. They provide the energy for the crowd.

In any system, there are the energetic sources, the other components that are influenced and in turn influence, and the uninvolved parts. The trick for treatment is to discover how to move the less-involved parts, continue to reduce the overall energy in the system, and to nudge the system toward lower noise and greater flexibility.

It may be said that our job is to reduce the noise in the above intersection: to increase the ease with which messages are exchanged in the brain. If we ask each person in the intersection to move, the ones that first move will be the ones least involved: the bystanders. With the bystanders absent, there is less encouragement for the collaborators and the instigators.

The next to move will be the least motivated of the collaborators. Their absence provides still less reinforcement for the more motivated collaborators and the instigators, making it easier to move more collaborators. In a reiterative

fashion, the crowd thins, with more collaborators losing motivation as it does. In the end, the instigators may or may not be moved. However, there is now much more room for traffic to flow and the intersection can be more functional. It is the function of the LENS map to empirically define which of the sites are bystanders, collaborators, and perhaps, the instigator(s)–the generators. Of course this is something of a conjecture and may to a large extent be unnecessary. However, it does provide a methodology for approaching the complex clinical pictures with which we deal. In fact, using the LENS map the way we do may be one of the factors contributing to the relatively short treatment times. There may well be alternative ways of organizing the treatment approach that could result in further reduction in treatment duration, more efficacious results, or both.

The Brain as a System. There are such things as simple problems. These cases generally have a sudden onset of symptoms without an inter-generational or genetic basis to the symptom. The treatments are even simpler for those people who were especially high functioning before their injury or trauma. Treatment of these individuals with acquired CNS problems is often a joy. They may be the cases shared among colleagues, the ones which impress the audiences, and propel the sales of EEG equipment. For these instances, it is quite plausible to apply traditional neurofeedback or the LENS method to one or two of the standard 10-20 electrode sites and watch the miracles happen. Unfortunately, informal surveys of therapists using all of the current models of neurofeedback equipment on the market evoke reports that from 50 to 80 percent of the time the therapists do not feel like they know what they are doing. They feel lost about treatment direction and disappointed at the results they are obtaining.

Achieving success with LENS at any one electrode site (i.e., reducing EEG amplitude and variability) can lead to behavioral rebounds and reactions such as transient hyperactivity or fatigue. When doing topographic maps sequentially at different electrode sites, it is quite apparent when the problems that a person has seem to be occurring within a system or multiple systems of activity as measured across the scalp. The complex cases invariably show many kinds of EEG activity (i.e., unwanted rises in amplitudes and variability) that are caused by isolated successes at the sites that were treated in isolation. If a site or a few sites are treated without recognition of the extant systems, then there are often untoward post-session problems.

This hypothesized activity occurring in systems may be the same as hypercoherence: the same frequency appearing at multiple sites across the scalp at the same time. If these sites are linked together, and if the therapist is treating one or a few of the sites, changes in those few sites will cause a reaction in the rest of the system which may both evoke strong concern or worry in the patient, and create management problems in treatment, as well as cause unnecessarily long and uneconomical treatment processes.

The topographic mapping process that we utilize holds promise to enable the therapist to understand how to approach the areas involved in the pathology in a graded, elegant way, and without any biases based on "known facts" stemming from neuropsychology or literature reports. Mapping reduces the chances that a statistically unusual site plays a prominent part in the functional pathology. It reduces the chance that the unusual site or combination of sites will be missed, delaying the problem's resolution.

The maps show the frequency bands' evoked amplitude undulations shrinking spatially, dampening, and eventually stabilizing in amplitude as treatment progresses. This translates into being able to observe the chaotic energy systems moving around and rearranging themselves across the scalp surface as they become electrically less noisy. The surface maps are transformed into other graphs that specify which sites are to be worked with, and in which sequence (see Figure 2).

Having these maps of evoked activity available also permits the therapist to compare current versus previously measured values. When there is too much of a discrepancy, the loss of accuracy indicates that the map is no longer a faithful guide to treatment and that another map is needed to accurately predict the strategic site sequences.

Sensitivity vs. Hypersensitivity. When patients first enter treatment they tend to see themselves as overly sensitive. In fact, they tend to be quite reactive, but quite insensitive. An ex-tremely reactive individual is so reactive to stimuli and caught up in the emotional, cognitive, glandular, vascular, immunological, and/or motoric elements of the reactions that there is literally no opening for being aware of the stimuli. Hypersensitive individuals are rarely aware of much about their situations or of their feelings. They are aware of their reactions to these situations and feelings, rather than of the situations themselves. For example, they may be overwhelmed by their reactions of discomfort, or overwhelmed by the difficulty of taking things in.

The LENS ordinarily reduces the amplitude and variability of the EEG across the spectrum. In other words, the EEG becomes less hyper-reactive to the LENS feedback. This may be a function of the enormous dynamic range of the feedback intensity, which can potentially be varied by 100,000 gradations from the weakest to most intense feedback intensity levels. Turning the feedback on and off will at times show correlated amplitude and variability changes in the EEG on the screen, even though patients cannot feel the feedback. As the patient's hyper-reactivity drops, the patient tends to experience a subjective increase in ease, greater ability to follow conversations, to understand what is read, and to think more clearly. Clarity is a reflection of greater perceptual acuity and a lessening of mental fog. Often there are reports of increasing quiescence and decreases in restlessness. The intersection, as in the above story, has become quieter and more functional. Another way to put it is that the patient is becoming more sensitive–but less hyper-reactive. The result is that the patient is more aware of the environment and of inner feelings; more aware of likes, dislikes, needs, and satisfactions of those needs. The good and bad news is that while the patient can be happier and unhappier, there is more chance, because of decreased hyper-reactivity, to be more thoughtful about life.

Sensitivity: Its Acknowledgment, Management, and Benefits. The phenomenon of sensitivity to feedback intensity is one of the most intriguing aspects of the LENS. There is an apparent relationship between dysfunction and reactivity to stimulation. Patients express this verbally and/or motorically. This can also be observed during treatment as increasing delta, theta, or alpha activity across a number of sites, without a return to baseline within five minutes. These factors led me and my colleagues to consider alternative treatment models arising from our new views regarding brain trauma and its resolution.

The apparent plasticity of the dysfunction under the feedback of the LENS itself casts considerable doubt on the traditionally held view that much post-trauma dysfunction is attributable to the trauma; perhaps it is largely attributable to the brain's own protective mechanisms. Rather than working with trauma-induced brain damage, in the case of brain injury we may need to be working with the brain's own self-protective neurochemical systems.

What is most important is that we apparently are far more sensitive than we have ever expected, at least when we become injured or in any way dysfunctional. Much of the medical establishment, and to a certain extent the psychological rehabilitation establishment, has taken up the "Jack LaLane" exercise, gain-through-pain approach to rehabilitation. This was the mentality which was originally applied to the LENS work until it was recognized that the opposite was the only approach that consistently produced positive outcomes. It has turned out that the more we take into account sensitivity, making treatment as gentle as possible in previously unimaginable ways, the neuronal strength of the patients has been supported, and recovery follows far more often than not.

This shift in paradigm regarding the units of analysis, intervention and mechanism of action often means that the feedback intensity is kept to a minimum. During the early sessions the therapist needs to know how to be content to make very small interventions until the patient, with decreased symptoms, becomes ready for more pungency in the feedback. It has only been when the patient's sensitivity has been carefully considered that maximum speed of treatment is achieved. Otherwise valuable treatment time is spent recovering from treatment-induced relapses.

Suppression. EEG activity suppression. Almost without exception, all relatively high amplitude EEG band activity drops (even with high beta) following LENS feedback. However, low amplitude and standard deviations can and do rise. When this occurs the low activity is understood to have been suppressed. Pre-

scription medication can cause this kind of suppression. Internal automatic self-medication with perhaps inhibitory neurotransmitters might also cause this kind of suppression.

At first it was thought that the rises in amplitude that occur with the LENS treatments were signs of over stimulation and signs of pathology. However, it has become apparent that most amplitude and standard deviation increases occur in the context of increasingly competent functioning–although not infrequently in the context of some narrowly defined and extremely disruptive symptoms. For example, while the patient is becoming more relaxed and less depressed, there may be an increase in seizures, tics, temper, muscular pain, toileting accidents, and perhaps substance abuse. These are not seen as side effects of treatment now. In contrast, they are now seen as transition states during which short-term compensations and inhibitions have been released. They occur in those with histories of the observed problems. It may be that the very problematic, potentially dangerous, and most likely socially very embarrassing symptoms were intuitively suppressed–and most likely forgotten, until the current treatment.

These symptoms, depending on their pathology and severity, typically last a week, and then remit. They may also re-occur when a virus, other infection, or other body change is still pre-clinical and unobserved. However, after one or two infection or bodily change cycles, they no longer appear.

It is extremely important that each prospective patient be interviewed for such previous historical symptoms. Their presence is not necessarily a contraindication for the LENS approach. But if they were present at one point in his or her life, it is a chance to ask the patient whether the symptoms for which he or she is seeking relief are important enough to out weigh the risk of re-encountering for a short time the intensely problematic symptoms from earlier life. It takes a relatively short while, during treatment, for the brain to integrate–rather than inhibit–problematic pathophysiology, and thus bring marked relief.

The What, Why, and How of the LENS. There are three considerations concerning the LENS and its mechanism: What is happening, why it happens, and what treatment strategies bring about the effect. These can be labeled, respectively: permeability, inhibitory neurotransmitter activity alterations, and applied chaos theory. The statements addressing each area of concern are testable.

What. Changes in cortical permeability: It has been observed that individuals with chronic central nervous system functioning problems have higher levels of recordable low frequency electrical activity at scalp sites. It has further been observed that as the functioning of the individual improves with treatment, the amplitude of the EEG diminishes across the spectrum at each scalp site.

On a descriptive level, the most parsimonious way to picture what happens as functioning improves and as the measured evoked EEG amplitude drops, might be in terms of decreasing permeability of the cortex: the higher amplitude activity probably remains present subcortically. It may be that it is simply not measurable at the scalp surface as the cortex re-assumes its integrative capacity and blocks the appearance of the higher amplitude subcortical activity at the surface. The use of indwelling (needle) electrodes at various depths simultaneously may help differentiate cortical from subcortical activity, and show with treatment, evidence of increased cortical activation as differentiated from subcortical activity.

Why. Inhibitory neurotransmitter activity alternations: Feeding back frequency information that is different from that which is measured, but nevertheless still a function of the frequency measured, may place different neurochemical demands on the synapses which feed the measured activity. If there is post-traumatic inhibitory neurotransmitter activity interfering with cortical function (i.e., making the cortex more permeable) and if the mechanism perpetuating this activity is disturbed and is altered, then the synaptic neurotransmitter mix might be altered to once again permit decreased permeability and proper cortical functioning.

How. Applied chaos therapy: Most neurofeedback treatment focuses on the shaping of activity in one or two frequency bands through voluntary controls at one or two sites. One of the complaints about the duration of neurofeedback treatment is that it takes too long and is too expensive. The sites commonly treated are, as often as not, the ones showing the highest measured amplitudes, making the task from the start a difficult one.

While treatment of acute patients with good premorbid histories may respond to a simpler treatment strategy, such a strategy may not suffice for patients with complicated, life-long histories and symptoms. In contrast, without trying to speed or slow the EEG activity, the LENS addresses all of the of the standard 10-20 system scalp sites as a method to control the feedback in a sequence based on a ranking of site-permeability (irritability) from least to most. By using this method, the activity at both the sites that have problems in isolation, and at sites that act in coherence systems, can be decreased in a predictable manner. This may reduce treatment time and expense in complicated cases, and increase the longevity of a positive outcome.

CONCLUSION

The LENS has shown significant effects in the treatment of a variety of CNS mediated disorders. Ongoing research will be required to fully understand the mechanisms of action and algorithms for directing treatment (e.g., site selection, feedback intensity, duration, etc.). The following are some tentative conclusions regarding the benefits and underlying principles of the LENS.

Treatment benefits include: decreased feelings of irritability, anger, fatigue, anxiety, depression, and decreased angina when caused by cortical problems. Improved mental clarity (decreased "mental fog"), sleep, energy, concentration, attention, short-term memory, improved vision and speech when due to cortical problems, and increased ease of functioning. Tangible clinical improvements are typically noted within three to six sessions. Reductions in EEG amplitude and variability will often be noted within the first five minutes of the first session.

The LENS in the Current Social/Scientific/ Clinical Context. The following are issues of concern expressed by non-The LENS professionals.

Invasiveness

In contrast to traditional EEG feedback, the LENS could be considered minimally invasive.

The field strength of the stimulation is only 10-18 watts/cm2, which is far less invasive than medication or electroconvulsive therapy, and microscopic in comparison to transcranial magnetic stimulation or even in comparison to the stimulation received from holding a cell phone to one's ear.

Other-Directed (Therapist Regulated) vs. Self-Regulation

Two attitudes are interwoven in this controversy. One idea is that consciousness is a requirement for self-regulation. If the regulation that occurs is not conscious and intentional, it is not self-regulation. Yet the spinal cord and lower brain centers are not only responsible for many of our life-support systems, but they also can learn and adapt quite nicely without conscious intervention. In other words, we may be just as smart subcortically (and unconsciously) as we are consciously. So it seems wasteful to devalue non-conscious self-regulation and to throw away resources that can be mobilized for learning and life enhancement. Furthermore, although conscious effort and work is involved with traditional neurofeedback, it is not so much teaching self-regulation as it is facilitating the operant conditioning of healthier brainwave patterns.

The second controversy is the locus of control issue, or who is in control, therapist or patient? This issue seems to be grounded in the naïve belief that traditional biofeedback places the patient in charge, and that he or she is truly engaged in self-regulation. There is, of course, the implication that when a therapist is administering an energy field, the process is controlled by the therapist. In fact, the design of the treatment protocol used in traditional biofeedback is also under therapist control (i.e., whether to enhance a particular high frequency activity and inhibit low frequency activity). Further, the operation of the threshold, which determines which EEG activity gets which kinds of reinforcement, is likewise under therapist control in traditional EEG biofeedback.

Similarly, the therapist is clearly in control of the structure of the LENS session, but is guided by the patient's subjective sense of what is comfortable and uncomfortable. In contrast, when using the LENS protocols, the goal of the LENS treatment is flexibility of neural functioning, and there is no unilateral influence on the brain to either produce more fast-wave activity or more slow-wave activity. The patient's brain is left free to do as it needs to, when it needs to, as the amplitude and variability decrease across the spectrum.

Hopefully, both LENS and general neurofeedback procedures will maximize the ability of the patient to be self-regulating. However, it is naive to hold the premise that traditional EEG biofeedback places the patient in charge of the structure of the treatment, or that neurofeedback is teaching self-regulation in the sense of learning a conscious skill. It seems that the more important scientific concern needs to be: Under which clinical conditions is LENS or traditional neurofeedback most effective and efficient? Each system may have its own domains of applicability.

Physical or Psychological Harm

The Thalidomide tragedy has made everyone aware of the importance of looking at long-term effects of a prospective treatment, and rightly so. It is always worth reviewing the probability that wherever there is change, there is disruption. And whether good or bad, there can always be unpleasant as well as beneficial effects, even if the treatment is "entirely natural." One issue here is not whether there are "unpleasant side effects," but to identify what they are. Side effects or adverse reactions have been noted with traditional neurofeedback technology (Hammond, Stockdale, Hoffman, Ayers, & Nash, 2001) and in fact, if misapplied traditional neurofeedback has the potential to evoke iatrogenic effects, including seizures (Lubar et al., 1981; Lubar & Shouse, 1976, 1977). Once identified, the prospective recipient of the treatment can weigh the benefits against the risks of treatment. The unpleasant side effects of treatment discovered to date echo the unpleasant effects of any other kind of change process, whether it is hypnosis, psychotherapy, biofeedback, yoga, etc. With the LENS system, no patient over the last three years has ever reported a new symptom; that is, one that had never before been experienced by that patient. However, any current symptom, physical or psychological, can be temporarily exacerbated.

Another issue here is to differentiate unpleasant "side-effects" from disruptive signs of health and recovery. As people become clearer about their own reactions to a difficult, unpleasant, and even treacherous world, they are inclined to become more angry, sad, or anxious, and appropriately so. They are apt to become less tolerant of what ought not to be tolerated. However, it is the amount of increased thoughtfulness and productivity about the noxious elements of life that makes these reactions different from the hyper-reactive, blind reactions that characterized their lives prior to the LENS treatment. These considerations need to be made clear when individuals are considering LENS treatment.

Dearth of Literature

It must be acknowledged that apart from this volume, there is only a limited scientific research (Donaldson, Sella, & Mueller, 1998; Mueller, Donaldson, Nelson & Layman, 2001; Schoenberger et al., 2001) on the use of LENS. We know little about the effects of variable-frequency feedback on EEG activity. However, we now have considerable clinical experience in working with a number of diagnoses. As with most clinical areas of application of traditional neurofeedback, adequately controlled outcome studies with LENS are lacking. Therefore, the informed consent process with patients must acknowledge these facts to allow patients to make an informed decision about using a more investigational treatment.

Fear of LENS Treatment Being Too Rapid

Finally we should mention a frequently expressed concern about the LENS producing therapist unemployment because it is too rapid or effective. It is true that the LENS often reduces treatment time, making for more rapid patient turnover, and placing new demands on a therapist's marketing skills. However, it also often increases a therapist's effectiveness, opens up treatment as an option to new populations, and makes treatment more affordable and enjoyable. Further, it increases the number of patients a therapist can help in shorter lengths of time.

Summary

LENS is an innovative type of neurofeedback that has evolved over the past 16 years. It involves the use of very weak electromagnetic energy fields which are fed back to the brain based on the brain's dominant frequency from moment-to-moment. This feedback is usually effective in reducing high amplitude activity, in many cases shortening the length of treatment that is required in comparison with traditional neurofeedback. Treatment sessions are brief, and because of the minimal demands it places on the patient it is very appealing to some patients and opens up treatment options for new populations of patients. The nature of LENS technology will also facilitate doing double-blind, placebo controlled studies which can advance our field.

NOTES

1. Some proportion of activity in the different frequency bands seems healthy, with either too much or too little being potentially problematic. Delta, for example, seems to have a functional role in facilitating inner concentration by suppressing extraneous cortical inputs. A delta deficit can correlate with reduced frontal cortical regulation or gating of maladaptive behavioral impulses or extraneous cues, and can be found in conditions such as cocaine addicts, alcoholics, ADD, subtypes of OCD, and schizophrenia (Alper, Prichep, Kowalek, Rosenthal, & John, 1998). Increased theta band activity may be seen in highly experienced mediators, and increased delta and theta EEG activity have also often been found in association with various kinds of cognitive activity, such as performing calculations (e.g., Fernandez et al., 1995; Klimesch, Doppelmayer, Russegger, & Pachinger, 1996).

2. Offsets were originally implemented to reduce the possibility of exacerbating seizure activity and EEG slowing. When amplitudes are unusually low, an offset of zero may help to stimulate the physiology to increase amplitude. However, we have very little experience to state this with any confidence.

REFERENCES

Alper, K. R., Prichep, L. S., Kowalek, S., Rosenthal, M. S., & John, E. R. (1998). Persistent QEEG abnormality in crack cocaine users at 6 months of drug abstinence. *Neuropsychopharmacology, 19* (1), 1-9.

Carter, J. L., & Russell, H. L. (1981). Changes in verbal performance of IQ discrepancy scores after left hemisphere EEG frequency control training. *American Journal of Clinical Biofeedback, 4*, 66-68.

Carter, J. L., & Russell, H. L. (1984). Application of biofeedback relaxation procedures to handicapped children: Final resort. (Project No. 443CH00207, Grant No. G008001608). Washington, DC: Bureau of Education for the Handicapped.

Carter, J. L., & Russell, H. L. (1993). A pilot investigation of auditory and visual entrainment of brain wave activity in learning disabled boys. *Texas Researcher, 4*, 65-73.

Davidson, R J., & Hydahl, K. H. (Eds.) (1996). *Brain asymmetry*. Cambridge, MA: Bradford Books, MIT Press.

Diamond, M. C. (1988). *Enriching heredity: The impact of the environment on the anatomy of the brain*. New York: The Free Press.

Donaldson, C. C. S., Sella, G. E., & Mueller, H. H. (1998). Fibromyalgia: A retrospective study of 252 consecutive referrals. *Canadian Journal of Clinical Medicine, 5* (6), 116-127.

Fernandez, T., Harmony, T., Rodriguez, M., Bernal, J., Silva, J., Reyes, A., et al. (1995). EEG activation patterns during the performance of tasks involving different components of mental calculation. *Electroencephalography & Clinical Neurophysiology, 94*, 175-182.

Gleick, J. (1988). *Chaos: Making a new science*. New York: Penguin

Hammond, D. C., Stockdale, S., Hoffman, D., Ayers, M. E., & Nash, J. (2001). Adverse reactions and potential iatrogenic effects in neurofeedback training. *Journal of Neurotherapy, 4* (4), 57-69.

Hughes, J. R., & John, E. R. (1999). Conventional and quantitative electroencephalography in psychiatry. *Journal of Neuropsychiatry and Clinical Neuroscience, 11*, 190.

Klimesch, W., Doppelmayer, M., Russegger, H., & Pachinger, T. (1996). Theta band power in the human scalp EEG and the encoding of new information. *NeuroReport, 7*, 1235-1240.

Lubar, J. L. (1985). Changing EEG activity through biofeedback applications for the diagnosis and treatment of learning disabled children. Theory into practice. *Ohio State University, 24*, 106-111.

Lubar, J. F., Shabsin, H. S., Natelson, S. E., Holder, G. S., Whitsett, S. F., Pamplin, W. E., et al. (1981). EEG operant conditioning in intractable epileptics. *Archives of Neurology, 38*, 700-704.

Lubar, J. F., & Shouse, M. N. (1976). EEG and behavioral changes in a hyperactive child concurrent with training of the sensorimotor rhythm (SMR): A preliminary report. *Biofeedback & Self-Regulation, 1* (3), 293-306.

Lubar, J. F., & Shouse, M. N. (1977). Use of biofeedback in the treatment of seizure disorders and hyperactivity. *Advances in Clinical Child Psychology, 1*, 204-251.

Mueller, H. H., Donaldson, C. C. S., Nelson, D. V., & Layman, M. (2001). Treatment of fibromyalgia incorporating EEG-driven stimulation: A clinical outcomes study. *Journal of Clinical Psychology, 57* (7), 933-952.

Niedermeyer, E., & da Silva, F. H. L. (Eds.) (1999). Electroencephalography: Basic principles, clinical applications, and related fields. Philadelphia, PA: Lippincott, Williams & Wilkins.

Ochs, L. (1995). *Many kinds of depression are curable*. http://www.flexyx.com/articles/deprcure.html

Peniston, E. G., & Kulkosky, P. J. (1991). Alpha-theta brainwave neurofeedback therapy for Vietnam veterans with combat-related posttraumatic stress disorder. *Medical Psychotherapy: An International Journal, 4*, 47-60.

Persinger, M. A. (Ed.) (1974). *ELF and VLF electromagnetic field effects*. New York: Plenum Press.

Quirk, J. A., Fish, D. R., Smith, S. J., Sander, J. W., Shorvon, S. D., & Allen, P. J. (1995). Incidence of photosensitive epilepsy: A prospective national study. *Electroencephalography & Clinical Neurophysiology, 95* (4), 260-267.

Rife, R. R. (1953). History of the development of a successful treatment for cancer and other virus, bacteria and fungi. San Diego: Rife Virus Microscope Institute.

Sandyk, R. (1994). Improvement in word-fluency performance in Parkinson's disease by administration of electromagnetic fields. *International Journal of Neuroscience, 77* (1-2), 23-46.

Schoenberger, N. E., Shiflett, S. C., Esty, M. L., Ochs, L., & Matheis, R. J. (2001). Flexyx neurotherapy system in the treatment of traumatic brain injury: An initial evaluation. *Journal of Head Trauma Rehabilitation, 16* (3), 260-274.

doi:10.1300/J184v10n02_02

APPENDIX A

This article seeks to offer some historical background, an outline of the theoretical basis for how the Low Energy Neurofeedback System (LENS) works, and the approach to treatment which is evolving from the applied clinical work and research being initiated by OchsLabs. The LENS is still evolving at a rapid pace. It is thus impractical to conceive of this overview as being up-to-date for any length of time. The reader is cautioned to avoid any conclusion that this information reflects current practice. The reader is also cautioned to avoid seeing any information presented herein as a claim for the LENS to be efficacious for any condition, medical or psychological. This is the most objective depiction possible of the evidence on hand for its benefits and risks. No claims are being made.

The reader is cautioned that the purpose of this article is to enumerate some of the phenomena, issues, and concerns which were encountered, and not to provide a decision tree about which settings, options, conditions, and choices are to be made in any particular clinical instance. The information about settings, conditions, and treatment options presented are to exemplify the concepts. The actual number of options and considerations in the treatment planning process are outside the scope of this article. Further, there is still not enough concrete research-based information about the particular benefits or drawbacks of any particular setting or settings, or whether such settings are useful or necessary. Component analyses are needed to determine which conditions (protocols) are necessary and useful.

The reader of this article may find more questions being raised than answered. This is the nature of the opening of a new arena of observation and study. In this case, this arena is the area of behavioral biophysics: the interaction of resonant (feedback) physical stimuli on brain functioning. It is possible to ask of most of the statements in this article, "What is the evidence?" "Where are the data?" In fact, after 15 years of this exploration there is still a search for the fundamental questions. Furthermore, after 15 years, how to do research with the LENS is only beginning to clarify itself.

APPENDIX B
CNS Functioning Assessment

Name _____ Date of Birth _____ Age _____

Today's Date _____ Time _____ Diagnosis _____

Are you able to drive a motor vehicle? Yes Partially No   **Are you able to work or study?**
Yes Partially No   **Are you able to sustain a close relationship with someone?** Yes Partially No

How frequently do you have problems in the following areas? Please pick a number from 0-to-10. "0" means *Not at all*, and "10" means *All the time*.

If one or more of your parents had this, or a similar problem, place a *P* in the column headed by "Parents?"

If the problem came on suddenly, put an *S* in the column head by "Suddenly?"

Sensory	Frequency (0-10)	Parents? Suddenly?
Light, in general, or lights, bother you	_____	_____
Problems with the sense of smell	_____	_____
Problems with vision	_____	_____
Problems with hearing	_____	_____
Problems with the sense of touch	_____	_____

Emotions		
Problems of sudden, unexplained changes in mood	_____	_____
Problems of sudden, unexplained fearfulness	_____	_____
Problems of unexplained spells of depression	_____	_____

Problems of unexplained spells of elation   _____   _____
Problems with explosiveness   _____   _____
Problems with irritability   _____   _____
Problems with suicidal thoughts or actions   _____   _____

Clarity

Feel "foggy" and have problems with clarity   _____   _____
Problems following conversations (with good hearing)   _____   _____
Problems with confusion   _____   _____
Problems following what you are reading   _____   _____
Realize you have no idea what you have been reading   _____   _____
Problems with concentration   _____   _____
Problems with attention   _____   _____
Problems with sequencing   _____   _____
Problems with prioritizing   _____   _____
Problems not finishing what you start   _____   _____
Problems organizing your room, office, paperwork   _____   _____
Problems with getting lost in daydreaming   _____   _____
You cover up that you don't know what was said or
   asked of you   _____   _____

Energy

Problems with stamina   _____   _____
Fatigue during the day   _____   _____
Trouble sleeping at night   _____   _____
Problems awakening at night   _____   _____
Problems falling asleep again   _____   _____

Memory

Forget what you have just heard   _____   _____
Forget what you are doing, what you need to do   _____   _____
Problems with procrastination and lack of initiative   _____   _____
Problems not learning from experience   _____   _____

Movement

Problems with paralysis of one or more limbs   _____   _____
Problems focusing or converging the eyes   _____   _____

Pain

Head pain that is steady   _____   _____
Head pain that is throbbing   _____   _____
Shoulder and neck pain   _____   _____
Wrist pain   _____   _____
Knee pain   _____   _____
All-over pain   _____   _____
Joint pain   _____   _____
Other pain (specify)   _____   _____

Other Problems

Problems with nausea   _____   _____
Skin problems   _____   _____
Problems with speech or articulation   _____   _____
Dizziness   _____   _____
Noise in ears (Tinnitus)   _____   _____

Treatment of Fibromyalgia Syndrome Using Low-Intensity Neurofeedback with the Flexyx Neurotherapy System: A Randomized Controlled Clinical Trial

Howard M. Kravitz, DO, MPH
Mary Lee Esty, PhD
Robert S. Katz, MD
Jan Fawcett, MD

SUMMARY. *Background.* Treatment of fibromyalgia syndrome (FMS) remains a clinical challenge. Pain, somatic and cognitive symptoms may be due to neurosensitization involving CNS-activated autonomic and musculoskeletal reactions, associated with EEG abnormalities that may respond to brainwave-based stimulation biofeedback. This study's objective was to examine the efficacy and safety of a novel EEG neurobiofeedback treatment, the Flexyx Neurotherapy System® (FNS), and electrophysiological responses in persons with fibromyalgia.

Methods. A randomized, double-blind, placebo-controlled clinical trial was conducted in two private practices: a free-standing neurobiofeedback center and a rheumatologist's office at an academic medical center. Sixty-four participants with FMS (American College of Rheumatology criteria; Wolfe et al., 1990) for at least three years and symptoms for at least 48 months with no recent remission were randomized to treatment. A total of 22 treatment sessions were administered over at least 11 weeks of active (n = 33) or sham (n = 31) FNS therapy. Primary efficacy measures were the Clinical Global Impressions improvement scores, Clinician (CGI-I) and Participant (PGI-I) versions. Secondary outcomes included dolorimetry and tender point count, questionnaires (fibromyalgia symptom scales, CNS Dysfunction Questionnaire, Fibromyalgia Impact Questionnaire, Symptom Checklist-90-R), and EEG activity (delta, alpha, total amplitude).

Results. More participants treated with active FNS than with sham improved partially or fully on the CGI-I at session 22 (p = .01) and follow-up (p = .04). The active FNS group had a higher

---

Howard M. Kravitz is affiliated with the Department of Psychiatry and the Department of Preventive Medicine, Rush University Medical Center, Chicago, IL.

Mary Lee Esty is affiliated with the Neurotherapy Center of Washington, Chevy Chase, MD.

Robert S. Katz is affiliated with the Department of Internal Medicine, Section of Rheumatology, Rush University Medical Center, Chicago, IL.

Jan Fawcett is affiliated with the Department of Psychiatry, University of New Mexico School of Medicine, Albuquerque, NM and the Department of Psychiatry, Rush University Medical Center, Chicago, IL.

Address correspondence to: Howard M. Kravitz, Rush University Medical Center, Department of Psychiatry, Marshall Field IV Building, 1720 West Polk Street, Chicago, IL 60612 (E-mail: hkravitz@rush.edu).

The authors thank the study staff at each site and all of the patients who participated in this research study. They also appreciate the diligent efforts of Ms. Mary Onofrio in organizing the data and assisting in database preparations.

This study was funded by the Delaney Foundation and an anonymous donor.

[Haworth co-indexing entry note]: "Treatment of Fibromyalgia Syndrome Using Low-Intensity Neurofeedback with the Flexyx Neurotherapy System: A Randomized Controlled Clinical Trial." Kravitz, Howard M. et al. Co-published simultaneously in *Journal of Neurotherapy* (The Haworth Medical Press, an imprint of The Haworth Press, Inc.) Vol. 10, No. 2/3, 2006, pp. 41-58; and: *LENS: The Low Energy Neurofeedback System* (ed: D. Corydon Hammond) The Haworth Medical Press, an imprint of The Haworth Press, Inc., 2006, pp. 41-58. Single or multiple copies of this article are available for a fee from The Haworth Document Delivery Service [1-800-HAWORTH, 9:00 a.m. - 5:00 p.m. (EST). E-mail address: docdelivery@haworthpress.com].

CGI-I full response rate at session 22 (p < .05) but not at one-week post-treatment (p = .07). Significant active versus sham PGI-I responses were not detected (p>.10). There was no significant treatment effect on any secondary outcome measure and no specific symptom improved preferentially with active compared with sham FNS. The most commonly reported side effect was fatigue/tiredness. Pre-treatment delta/alpha EEG amplitude ratio > 1 was associated with PGI-I (but not CGI-I) response independent of treatment group assignment.

Conclusion. FNS monotherapy is insufficient for treating chronic, nonremitting FMS. doi:10.1300/J184v10n02_03 *[Article copies available for a fee from The Haworth Document Delivery Service: 1-800-HAWORTH. E-mail address: <docdelivery@haworthpress.com> Website: <http://www.HaworthPress.com> © 2006 by The Haworth Press, Inc. All rights reserved.]*

KEYWORDS. Fibromyalgia, Flexyx Neurotherapy System, neurofeedback, controlled clinical trial, treatment

INTRODUCTION

Fibromyalgia is a syndrome of unknown etiology and uncertain pathophysiology (Simms, 1994). Fibromyalgia syndrome (FMS) is characterized primarily by widespread pain, decreased pain threshold, diffuse tenderness, sleep disturbance, fatigue, and often psychological distress (Forseth, Gran, Husby & Forre, 1999; Lawrence et al., 1998; Makela, 1999; McBeth, Macfarlane, Hunt, & Silman, 2001). Diagnosed using the American College of Rheumatology's (ACR) criteria (Wolfe et al., 1990), this condition is more prevalent in women than in men across the entire adult age spectrum (Wolfe, Ross, Anderson & Russell, 1995; Wolfe, Ross, Anderson, Russell & Hebert, 1995). Disability due to FMS is a major public health concern due to impaired functioning in occupational, social and family roles, reduced quality of life, and increased health services utilization (Burckhardt, Clark, & Bennett, 1993; Calahan & Blalock, 1997; White & Harth, 1999; White, Speechley, Harth, & Ostbye, 1999; Wolfe & Vancouver Fibromyalgia Consensus Group, 1996).

A clinical diagnosis of FMS requires widespread pain for at least three month's duration. Decreased pain threshold is elicited by direct digital palpation of specific sites called tender points (Wolfe & Cathey, 1985) and with a pressure algometer (dolorimeter) (Simms, Goldenberg, Felson, & Mason, 1988; Tunks, Crook, Norman, & Kalaher, 1988). ACR criteria define "widespread" as pain on palpation of at least 11 of 18 designated tender point sites (Wolfe et al., 1990).

Treatment of FMS remains a clinical challenge. In a meta-analysis of 49 short-term clinical trials (one week to six months) involving 2,066 participants, Rossy et al. (1999) found that many pharmacological and non-pharmacological treatments benefited persons with FMS. In controlled studies, non-pharmacological treatment was more efficacious than pharmacological treatment alone in improving self-report of FMS symptoms (e.g., pain, fatigue, morning stiffness) and a similar trend for improvement was found on daily functioning measures. However, improvement in daily functioning consistently showed the lowest effect size in both pharmacological and non-pharmacological studies. Moderately large effect sizes were found for improved physical and psychological status but comparisons with pharmacological treatments showed no differential effect. There were significant benefits for non-pharmacological treatment with and without concurrent medication use.

Biofeedback is one non-pharmacological modality. Biofeedback treatment, particularly electromyography biofeedback using surface electromyography (sEMG) procedures, show mixed results (Rossy et al., 1999; Schwartz, 1995; Simms, 1994). Donaldson, Nelson and Schulz (1998), Mueller, Donaldson, Nelson and Lyman (2001), and Flor, Birbaumer, and Turk (1990) suggested that the characteristic FMS neurosomatic symptoms (e.g., cognitive, mood, sleep) may be due to a neurosensitization process that becomes self-perpetuating through CNS-activated autonomic and musculoskeletal reactions, resulting in muscle ischemia and hypoxia and the release of pain-producing substances in the periphery that feedback to the CNS. Thus, tender point abnormalities may represent secondary hyperalgesia, which depends on central nervous system pain mechanisms (Staud, 2002). The outcome of this process may be a chronic generalized pain syndrome that is associated with EEG abnormalities and that may respond (i.e., by "CNS desensitization") to a brainwave-based biofeedback known as EEG biofeedback or neurofeedback (Budzynski, 1999; Mueller et al., 2001).

Mueller et al. (2001) treated a preliminary series of thirty patients primarily (n = 26) or exclusively (n = 4) with EEG-driven stimulation (EDS), a specific form of neurofeedback, and reported that a variety of FMS symptoms improved substantially. Treatment endpoint in this case series was self-reported "noticeable improvements in mental clarity, mood, and sleep" and change from diffuse to localized pain (Mueller et al., 2001, p. 933). Thus it is not surprising that they found "significant reductions in a broad array of symptomatology" (p. 947). Patients were treated until they responded, at a cost of approximately $3,500 to $4,500 for assessment and treatment. EDS treatment ranged from 16 to 80 hours (mean = 37 hours) spread over 5 to 36 weeks (mean = 15 weeks). Most patients received additional therapies including sEMG biofeedback, physical therapy, massage therapy, and medication.

In this study we investigated the use of the Flexyx Neurotherapy System® device (FNS; Flexyx, LLC, Walnut Creek, CA). Similar to EDS, which is described as an "interactive EEG entrainment device" that uses a combination of EEG biofeedback and frequency-modulated light stimulation that is fed back to the patient to entrain the EEG (Mueller et al., 2001), FNS combines conventional EEG biofeedback and subthreshold photic stimulation (see Ochs commentary in this volume) in an effort to change EEG patterns (Schoenberger, Shiflett, Esty, Ochs, & Matheis, 2001). Initially, FNS was developed for altering EEG patterns associated with cognitive dysfunction and ultimately to improve functioning in persons with traumatic brain injury (Schoenberger et al., 2001). FNS does not require the subject's attention, focus, or orienting toward the feedback because the stimulus is not perceptible. Instead,

the feedback signal is thought to affect tissues of the brain and related structures in some as yet mechanistically undefined way without the subject's conscious participation (Len Ochs, personal communication, July 17, 1999). FNS's potential benefit in fibromyalgia has been shown only in the described uncontrolled case series. The most common side effects have been fatigue, anxiety, hyperactivity, and a temporary intensification of symptoms that previously had been problematic (Len Ochs, personal communication, July 17, 1999; Schoenberger et al., 2001). These reactions usually resolved within hours or days following temporary withdrawal from and/or decreased exposure to the feedback, and may have been due to over-treatment.

We conducted what is, to our knowledge, the first randomized, double-blind, placebo-controlled study to assess the efficacy and safety of FNS neurofeedback for short-term (22 sessions; 2 sessions/week for 11 weeks) treatment of patients with FMS.

METHODS

Participants

Outpatients were recruited to the study at two private practice sites, a free-standing neuro-biofeedback center in Chevy Chase, MD and a rheumatologist's office located at an academic medical center in Chicago, IL. The Chevy Chase site also recruited via newspaper advertisements and at a public meeting of the local Fibromyalgia Association. Initially, a third site was involved but due to alleged protocol violations and concerns regarding data integrity this site was dropped about midway through its enrollment; data for these participants were not available for analysis. Dr. Len Ochs, developer of the FNS equipment, coordinated research activity at all sites. The Chicago site handled administrative activities and data management. Each study site obtained local institutional review board approval of the protocol. Participants gave written informed consent at screening and were not paid for participating.

Enrollment occurred between September 1999 and June 2001. Selection criteria included: (a) age 18-62 years old; (b) diagnosed with fibromyalgia by ACR criteria (Wolfe et al., 1990) at least three years before study entry, by a rheumatologist or appropriate specialist; (c) experienced symptoms for at least 48 months with no recent remission of symptoms to any degree; (d) free of chronic viral infection; (e) no history of any significant medical conditions such as hepatitis, herpes, lupus, multiple sclerosis, rheumatoid arthritis, polio, epilepsy, rheumatic fever, or cancer, whether a current condition or in remission; (f) free of any condition contributing to medical instability, such as any history of seizures, asthma, diabetes, hypotension; (g) no history of neck or back surgeries; (h) no multiple chemical sensitivities; (i) no history of debilitating chronic fatigue; (j) free of developmental disabilities, or significant psychological disorder for which treatment has become necessary, or history of electroconvulsive therapy; (k) not currently taking morphine or its derivatives (e.g., oxycontin), benzodiazepines, or fluoxetine; (l) not presently engaged in litigation regarding their physical condition; (m) no prior exposure to the study treatment; (n) attained a minimum educational level of grade 8; and (o) able to read and comprehend English. Those meeting these criteria were invited to a screening evaluation that included dolorimetry and EEG mapping (described below) to determine eligibility. Screening laboratory tests (blood and urine) were done to rule out any significant medical problems that could contribute to symptoms of fibromyalgia or widespread pain.

Procedures

Study Treatment

Based on previous clinical experience, treatment sessions were scheduled twice weekly for eleven weeks. The necessary equipment for EEG neurofeedback consists of (a) a 486 DX2-66 MHz personal computer with 8 megabytes of RAM, 1 gigabyte hard drive, tape backup, 2 serial-I parallel input/output ports, 16550 UART, S-VGA capability, a monitor and mouse, and capable of running Windows 3.1 or Windows 95; (b) J&J Enterprises 1-330 Compact 2-channel EEG with an on-board feedback generator powering; (c) J&J Enterprises goggles, which include diodes embedded in a set of plastic glasses; (d) a set of J&J goggles modified to be incapable of providing any feedback; and (e) Flexyx USE-2 Software and Microsoft Word 6/Excel 5 or MS Office 4.2. The Flexyx USE2 software was written specifically for this system and is not available commercially. The equipment has been described elsewhere (Mueller et al., 2001; Ochs, 1993, 1997; Schoenberger et al., 2001). MLE and LO trained the FNS therapists.

Prior to randomization, participants were required to demonstrate an average delta EEG amplitude of at least 3.0 microvolts with a standard deviation of at least 0.70 on the EEG map. These criteria are based upon clinical traumatic brain injury data (Schoenberger et al., 2001). Brain stem damage is reflected in suppressed amplitudes and this baseline was established to assess the presence of dysfunction while still allowing for the effect of medications.

Data from the FNS screening/mapping session provided the treatment guide for the active/sham FNS treatment sessions. This screening session of topographic EEG assessment was conducted without any feedback component. FNS maps were done under medication conditions requiring that all pain and antidepressant medications that can be safely stopped not be taken for 48 hours prior to mapping. The importance of this mapping procedure is that it generates a critical path specifying the sequence in which one 10-20 site is to be designated as the "active" site from which to measure the EEG during treatment and determines the sequence in which sites are treated. The EEG is monitored for four seconds at each of 21 electrode sites. The electrical activity at this so-designated site controls the pulsation frequency of the feedback.

Eligible participants were randomly assigned to one of the two treatment conditions, either active EEG neurofeedback (active FNS) or a placebo condition (sham FNS), in which all aspects of treatment were identical except that no feedback was given. All participants wore identical-appearing goggles/glasses during the treatment. Although very small electromagnetic pulses may have been delivered through the electrode wires, the sham FNS goggles/glasses should not have provided sufficient electrical input to provide feedback. A dipole switch was added to prevent any stimulation from reaching the electrode wires before treating the final 29 participants (13 of whom received sham FNS). Separate analyses of this subgroup showed no significant increases in active versus sham FNS treatment response differences so all participants were combined in the analyses. Goggles/glasses were coded by the manufacturer and were assigned to each research site by a third party. We considered the sham (placebo) condition credible because the intensity of feedback in the treatment condition is too low to be perceived visually. Strobing of the diodes could not be perceived by participants in either condition. Double-blinding of both therapists and participants was maintained until after the first follow-up assessment evaluation, one week post-treatment.

During FNS treatment sessions, active and sham, the participants sat comfortably with their eyes closed, engaged in no specific activity, with the glasses held by the therapist so that the ear pieces did not block the diodes, and their ends two inches from the participant's cheeks. The feedback intensity was .001 during all phases of the treatment. Feedback sessions provided for a minimum of one second and a maximum of three seconds per session. A maximum number of three sites were treated during a session. If a participant could not tolerate three seconds per session (i.e., reporting treatment-related discomfort during the session or within the subsequent 24 hours) further reduction in intensity was achieved by holding the glasses up to twenty inches from the participant's face.

Participants were permitted to continue stable doses of medications during the study. Without permitting this, we could not have enrolled subjects in this study; few participants were willing (or thought they would be able) to stop pain or sleep medications, including psychotropics, despite their apparent ineffectiveness (Scharf, 2003). However, pain medications, psychotropics, and anti-inflammatory medications had to be stopped for at least 48 hours before FNS maps (as described above). During treatment, medication doses could be reduced if indicated but not raised, and new medications except for those unrelated to fibromyalgia treatment (e.g., antibiotics, anti-sinus medication) could not be started.

Randomization

The randomization schedule was obtained from a website (http://www.randomizer.org; June 12, 2006) and was distributed in separate blocks of eight to each site. The randomization ratio varied within each block (i.e., not necessarily 4:4) but an overall 1:1 study ratio of active FNS to sham treatment was planned. Blocks of eight were allocated so that treatment could be unblinded after participants completed the one-week follow-up evaluation and sham FNS nonresponders could be offered an opportunity to repeat the 22-session treatment protocol with open-label active FNS soon after completing the blinded trial. Non-varying and equal (4:4) ratios would allow therapists to determine the treatment allocation sequence because they also administered the open-label treatment.

Measurements

Selecting a single primary outcome measurement that adequately characterizes the FMS treatment response is challenging because there are a number of different aspects. Persons may respond to treatment in diverse ways and FNS could have a variety of effects. Therefore several outcome measurement instruments, each examining a different main domain of symptom(s) and/or function, were used.

Clinical Global Impression

The Clinical Global Impressions Scale (Guy, 1976) global improvement scales, clinician- (CGI-I) and participant- (PGI-I) rated versions, were the primary outcome measures. Although there is no generally accepted and reliable measurement for gauging severity or change in FMS symptoms this instrument is used extensively in clinical trials. White and Harth (1996) reviewed outcome measures used in clinical trials for FMS and found that the most sensitive indicator of change was the physician's global assessment. Physician global assessment score as measured by visual analog scale also was a component of Simms, Felson and Goldenberg's (1991) three-item response criteria set.

A rating of 1 (very much improved) or 2 (much improved) on the CGI-I and PGI-I 7-point scales is considered a full response ("remission"). The clinician-rated severity of illness (CGI-S) subscale ranges from 1 (normal, not at all symptomatic) to 7 (among the most extremely symptomatic patients) and was rated prior to the first treatment session.

Dolorimetry and Tender Point Counts

Dolorimetry is a procedure for quantitatively assessing pain tolerance/threshold over hypersensitive areas. The dolorimeter used was a hand-held spring-loaded gauge with a range of 0-10 kg and capped with a 1.54 cm^2 stopper (pressure threshold meter; Pain Diagnostics and Treatment, Inc., Great Neck, NY). Dolorimetry was performed at the 18 sites delineated in the ACR criteria for fibromyalgia (Wolfe et al., 1990). Those performing this procedure, masters-level trained rheumatology nurse-practitioners in Chicago and trained non-medical research assistants in Chevy Chase, were taught to increase the dolorimeter pressure at a consistent rate of (approximately) 1 kg/second and to record the pressure at which participants reported pain, not tenderness. A mean dolorimetry score was calculated at each assessment by summing measurements from each of the 18 anatomic sites. To reduce the skew of the data, the maximum score recorded at each dolorimetry site was 4 kg/1.54 cm^2. Dolorimetry was repeated at sessions 9, 16, 22 and post-treatment follow-up. Inter-rater reliability data between sites were not obtained.

Tender point counts were based on dolorimetry data. Instead of conducting independent tender point examinations, each dolorimetry-elicited positive site was counted as a tender point. Thus, a "positive" tender point was defined as pain elicited by pressure less than 4 kg/1.54 cm^2 at a dolorimetry site. At study entry, this criterion level of pain had to be present in at least 11 of the 18 ACR criteria-defined sites.

Fibromyalgia Symptom Scales

Participants completed seven Likert-type scales measuring pain (generalized and specific), "fibro-fog" (memory, concentration, multitasking; Donaldson, Sella & Mueller,

1998), depression, and fatigue, before starting treatment and at sessions 5, 9, 13, 16, 19, 22 and at follow-up. For each symptom, participants were instructed to rate its severity over the preceding seven days (including the session day) on a horizontal scale ranging from 1 ("none") to 10 ("extremely severe").

Symptom Checklist-90-R (SCl-90-R)

Psychological factors were measured with the SCL-90-R (Derogatis, 1994), a multidimensional, self-report symptom inventory. The two treatment groups were compared on the three global indices of the overall extent of psychological distress. The Global Severity Index is a mean of all items. The Positive Symptom Total and Positive Symptom Distress Index scores are based on all items endorsed as "not at all" responses. Higher scores indicate more severe symptoms. The SCL-90-R was administered at screening and one-week post-treatment.

Fibromyalgia Impact Questionnaire (FIQ)

The FIQ (Burckhardt, Clark & Bennett, 1991) is a brief, self-rated multidimensional instrument for assessing symptoms, functioning and health status. The time frame is the last seven days. The modified version that we used included a question regarding number of days slept well and a checklist of symptoms experienced in the previous three months. Also, we used horizontal Likert-type scales, similar to the specific fibromyalgia symptom scales and ranging from 0 (no problem/symptom absent) to 9 (symptom very severe), instead of the visual analog scales. The FIQ was administered at screening and one-week post-treatment.

CNS Dysfunction Questionnaire (Flexyx, LLC, 1996)

This instrument consists of eight subscales–sensory, emotions, clarity, energy, memory, movement, pain, and "other problems." It was completed pre-treatment and was repeated at sessions 9, 16, and 22. The principal focus was to assess cognitive concerns ("fibro-fog") which are reported commonly by patients with fibromyalgia. Subscales have 2 to 13 items each, which are rated on frequency of occurrence from 0 (not at all) to 10 (all the time); the total score is obtained by summing the subscale scores.

Side Effects

Side effects were monitored at each session by asking participants if they had experienced any problems or symptoms. These were graded as 0, none; 1, does not significantly interfere with functioning; 2, significantly interferes with functioning; 3, nullifies therapeutic effect.

Data Analysis

Baseline characteristics were summarized for the whole sample and by treatment group assignment. Categorical variables were compared using chi-square or Fisher's exact test for count data and continuous variables were compared using independent t-tests for means.

Outcome assessments were conducted prior to that session's treatment. Thus, session 1 baseline assessments were conducted after randomization but before the first treatment, and the final on-treatment assessment, which was conducted at session 22, was completed prior to the final treatment. The one-week post-treatment outcomes were conducted after a week of no treatment to assess continued efficacy. Because the purpose of this report is to present acute treatment effects, we are interested mainly in the session 22 response, but for comparison we also report the one-week post-treatment outcomes. Symptom worsening at this follow-up could be due to treatment discontinuation effects and/or loss of supportive contact with staff.

The primary efficacy measure was the proportion achieving full response on the CGI-I and PGI-I scales. Dropping the third study site reduced the expected total enrollment to 64 participants for the two remaining sites. With 32 per treatment group, the power to detect a true active versus sham treatment difference in response rates is .73, based on a predicted 30% difference in percentages of CGI-I responders.

Active versus sham treatment response based on dichotomized end-of-treatment global improvement scores was analyzed using multivariate logistic regression (Hosmer & Lemeshow, 2000) for the last available assessment point (last observation carried forward). Baseline covariates in these models included pre-treatment CGI-S in the CGI-I analysis, and PGI-I since the initial screening score for the PGI-I analysis.

Secondary outcomes included two pain measures (dolorimetry, tender point counts), and four self-report clinical scales (symptom scales, CNS Dysfunction Questionnaire, SCL-90-R distress scales, FIQ). Repeated measures analyses for data collected at more than two time points (including pre-treatment) were conducted using the generalized estimating equation approach (GEE; Diggle, Heagerty, Liang, & Zeger, 2002). GEE models the mean response as a function of time within each treatment group and adjusts for within-site correlations of outcome measures (since subjects within a single site are more likely to be similar). This approach also permits inclusion of subjects with missing data so that subjects may contribute different numbers of observations. Pre-treatment baseline score for the outcome measure was a covariate. Outcomes measured only twice, pre-treatment and end of treatment (either session 22 or one-week post-treatment), were analyzed using repeated measures analysis of covariance. Differential improvement in the active FNS group versus the sham group was assessed by the treatment group-by-session (time) interaction, the statistical test of primary interest. Clinical site (Chevy Chase, Chicago) and its interactions with treatment and time were included in the models. If any site interaction term was statistically significant, treatment effect was re-estimated using only the Chevy Chase sample since most participants were treated there. If all site interaction terms were statistically non-significant they were omitted and the site was retained as a covariate. Safety data are presented according to randomization assignment.

Evoked EEG amplitudes (mean, standard deviation), in microvolts of delta, alpha, and total activity, were obtained before treatment was administered and at sessions 9, 16 and 22. We determined whether the baseline minus endpoint (session 22) amplitude differed between the two treatment groups. CGI-I and PGI-I responses at session 22 were examined as a function of pre-treatment minus session 22 change in EEG amplitude means and standard deviations to see if treatment outcome was related to EEG change. Finally, we explored whether the global impressions outcomes were related to relative EEG amplitudes (i.e., ratios; Laibow, 1999). We expected better responses if the pre-treatment delta mean amplitude was greater than the alpha mean amplitude (i.e., delta/alpha ratio > 1).

Statistical analyses were conducted using the Statistical Package for the Social Sciences (SPSS for Windows Release 6.1.3, SPSS Inc., Chicago, IL, 1995) and Stata (Stata Release 7.0, Stata Corp., College Station, TX, 2001). Data are presented as frequency counts, percentages, and mean ± 1 sd, unless otherwise specified. Alpha level was set to 0.05 for statistical significance and results are reported as two-tailed tests of hypotheses unless otherwise specified. As described above, multiple symptom-related outcomes were analyzed because of uncertainty regarding the specific outcome measure(s) that FNS might affect. P values from secondary outcome measures were interpreted as descriptive in nature. To avoid possible Type II errors we did not adjust for multiple comparisons (Rothman, 1990).

RESULTS

Recruitment and Retention

Of 159 screened for eligibility (24 in Chicago, 135 in Chevy Chase), 64 (40%) participants met entry criteria and were randomized to treatment (8 [33%] in Chicago, 56 [41%] in Chevy Chase), 33 to active FNS and 31 to sham FNS treatment, and 58 (90.6%) completed all 22 treatment sessions (30 active, 28 sham). Five participants (3 sham, 2 active), all from the Chevy Chase site, did not complete at least one post-randomization efficacy evaluation and were excluded from the treatment outcome analyses. Reasons for discontinuance included an extended trip abroad, preferred taking medication, long commute to treatment sessions, family emergency, and job change that interfered with scheduling treatment sessions. No participant dropped out due to treatment-related side effects. One Chevy Chase participant

dropped out after treatment session 14 due to intercurrent illness unrelated to FNS treatment. Last available data for this participant, who was randomized to active treatment, were carried forward in the endpoint CGI-I and PGI-I analyses. GEE analyses were based on the treated sample of 59. Treatment outcome data collected only at session 22 and/or one-week post-treatment could be analyzed only for the 58 study completers.

Pre-Treatment Baseline

Sample Characteristics

Table 1 shows the baseline comparisons for the two treatment groups. Participants ranged in age from 21-62 years old, and were mainly well-educated, middle-aged married women. Most (43; 67.2%) were employed. On average, participants reported that their symptoms began over a decade before study entry and that they were first treated for these symptoms approximately one to three years after symptom onset. However, they were not diagnosed with fibromyalgia until two to five and one-half years later. Most commonly, the onset of fibromyalgia symptoms was attributed to physical trauma (e.g., accident or injury) or some other or unknown cause. Thirteen percent reported a family history of fibromyalgia. The two treatment groups were comparable on all of these characteristics.

Medication Use

Participants randomized to active FNS reported using at least one more type of medication at study entry than those randomized to sham treatment. However, Table 1 shows that the two treatment groups differed only in use of allergy medication/decongestants. Vitamins (79.7%), pain medications (71.9%; persons using opioids were excluded), and psychotropics (64.1%; particularly antidepressants and hypnotics) were the most frequently used medications. Reproductive hormone therapies were used by 34.4% (hormone replacement or oral contraceptive), herbals or dietary supplements or homeopathic remedies by 25%, and muscle relaxants by 18.8%. No other type of medication was used by at least 10% of the sample.

TABLE 1. Baseline Characteristics of Whole Sample and Each Treatment Group

	All Participants	FNS Treatment	Sham Treatment	P value[b]
Number of participants	64	33[a]	31[a]	
Site, number (%)				.71
Chevy Chase, MD	56 (88)	28 (85)	28 (90)	
Chicago, IL	8 (13)	5 (15)	3 (10)	
Age in years, mean (sd)	46.9 (9.2)	45.9 (9.5)	48.1 (8.9)	.35
Gender, number (%) female	59 (92)	30 (91)	29 (94)	1.00
Race/Ethnicity, number (%)				.67[c]
White	59 (92)	31 (94)	28 (90)	
Marital status, number (%)				.43[d]
Married	39 (61)	18 (55)	21 (68)	
Single	18 (28)	10 (30)	8 (26)	
Divorced	7 (11)	5 (15)	2 (6)	
Education in years, mean (sd)	16.3 (2.4)	16.5 (2.5)	16.2 (2.2)	.62
Years since symptom onset, Mean (sd)	11.3 (8.1) (n = 63)	11.4 (8.2) (n = 32)	11.2 (8.1)	.89
Years since diagnosed, Mean (sd)	5.6 (3.2) (n = 63)	5.1 (2.6) (n = 32)	6.2 (3.6)	.15
Years since first treatment, Mean (sd)	9.5 (6.7) (n = 62)	10.6 (7.6) (n = 32)	8.3 (5.4) (n = 30)	.17
Precipitant, number (%)				.95
Post-infection	6 (9)	3 (9)	3 (10)	
Physical trauma	25 (39)	14 (42)	11 (36)	
Infection & trauma	8 (13)	4 (12)	4 (13)	
Other/Unknown	25 (39)	12 (36)	13 (42)	
Family history FMS, number (%)	8 (13)	4 (12)	4 (13)	1.00
Medication groups, mean (sd, Range) [Total = 27]	4.0 (1.9) (1-9)	4.6 (1.9)	3.4 (1.7)	.01
Allergy/Decongestant Medication, number (%)	9 (14)	8 (24)	1 (3)	.03
CGI[e] severity, mean (sd, range)	4.7 (1.1, 3-7)	4.7 (1.1)	4.7 (1.1)	.27
PGI,[f] visit 1, mean (sd, range)	4.2 (0.9, 2-7)	4.3 (1.1)	4.1 (0.7)	.30
Tender points, mean (sd, range)	16.8 (2.0, 11-18)	16.8 (2.3)	16.8 (1.8)	.51
Dolorimetry, mean (sd, range)	1.6 (0.9, 0-3.5)	1.5 (1.0)	1.7 (0.9)	.23

[a] Two participants in the Flexyx Neurotherapy System (FNS) treatment group and 3 subjects in the sham treatment group, all from the Chevy Chase site, dropped out of the study before completing at least one post-treatment assessment and were not included in the outcome analyses. Columns may not sum to 100% due to rounding.
[b] Based on chi-square or Fisher's exact test for count data and on t-test for comparing means.
[c] Comparison of white versus minorities (1 African-American and 1 Hispanic in FNS group, and 2 Hispanics and 1 "Other" in sham group).
[d] Comparison of married versus unpartnered (single, divorced), chi-square test p = .41.
[e] Clinician's Global Impressions, severity of fibromyalgia (FMS) illness at screening.
[f] Patient's Global Impressions, how felt since initial screen.

During the treatment trial, 11 participants (8 sham, 3 active FNS) decreased their pain and/or psychotropic medication ($\chi^2 = 2.33$, df = 1, p = .13).

Clinical Severity

The two treatment groups were comparably symptomatic on the screening CGI-S scale (mean = 4.7; moderately to markedly symptomatic). The two treatment groups also had similar mean dolorimetry (1.5-1.7 kg/1.54 cm² and positive tender point (mean = 16.8) scores, indicating marked tenderness. At the first session (before treatment), the active FNS group was slightly but significantly more severely symptomatic on CGI-S change score (active = 4.9, sham = 4.5; t = 2.47, df = 62, p = .016), and the mean PGI (active = 4.3, sham = 4.1) indicated "no change" since screening.

Site Differences

Pre-treatment global impressions and dolorimetry scores differed significantly at the two sites. The Chicago sample was less severely symptomatic than the Chevy Chase sample on the CGI-S (screen, 3.6 ± 0.5 versus 4.9 ± 1.0, p = .001; session 1, 3.9 ± 1.0 versus 4.9 ± 1.1, p < .02) but not on the PGI. Screening dolorimetry was 2.8 ± 0.5 in Chicago and 1.4 ± 0.8 in Chevy Chase, and tender point scores were 14.0 ± 3.0 in Chicago and 17.2 ± 1.5 in Chevy Chase (both p < .0005).

Treatment Outcomes

Primary Outcomes–Global Measures (CGI and PGI)

As shown in Table 2, there were notable differences in the active FNS group response rates measured with these two scales. In multivariate logistic regression analyses, controlling for baseline severity and treatment site, active treatment was associated with a higher improvement rate according to the CGI-I at session 22 (Wald test = 3.91, df = 1, p < .05). At one-week post-treatment, there was only a non-significant trend for a treatment group difference (Wald test = 3.18, df = 1, p = .07). There were no significant treatment group differences in PGI-I scores at either session 22 or at one-week post-treatment.

TABLE 2. Summary of Treatment Outcomes–Global Impressions Improvement at Final Session and One-Week Post-Treatment[a]

	Session 22		One Week Post-Treatment		P Value[b]	
	FNS	Sham	FNS	Sham	Pre-22	Pre-1-Week Post
	(n = 31)	(n = 28)	(n = 31)	(n = 28)		
CGI-I, n (%)[c]	15 (48)	7 (25)	15 (48)	8 (29)	.05	.07
PGI-I, n (%)[c]	7 (23)	8 (29)	8 (26)	6 (21)	.75	.56

[a] FNS, Flexyx Neurotherapy System®; CGI-I, clinician's global impressions improvement score; PGI-I, participant's global impressions improvement score. CGI-I and PGI-I rated in reference to change since began treatment.

[b] P value for each global impressions improvement score (CGI-I, PGI-I) is based on logistic regression model estimates using the Wald test statistic with one degree of freedom for the treatment effect, adjusted for site and baseline score (CGI-I analysis is adjusted for baseline CGI severity score because CGI-I is not measured at baseline; PGI-I analysis is adjusted for baseline self-reported improvement since screening visit. In all analyses the treatment-by-site interaction term was dropped because it was statistically non-significant. Last observation was carried forward for one FNS-treated subject who dropped out after session 13.

[c] Number (%) rated 'very much' or 'much' improved.

Participants also were categorized according to therapists' ratings of therapeutic effect taking into account partial responses (moderate/marked versus minimal/no change/worse). At session 22, active FNS was rated as having a moderate to marked effect for 56.7% and sham FNS was rated as having a moderate to marked effect for 25%; one-week post-treatment, active and sham FNS were rated as effective for 50% and 25%, respectively. Controlling for baseline symptom severity, active FNS was rated as having a greater therapeutic effect than the sham therapy at session 22 (Wald test = 6.14, df = 1, p = .01) and one-week post-treatment (Wald test = 4.09, df = 1, p = .04).

Secondary Outcomes–Pain and Other Symptom Measurements

Dolorimetry. Table 3 shows that the pain threshold in the FNS treatment group improved minimally through session 22 and at one-week post-treatment follow-up. Differential improvement was not observed between the active and sham FNS groups. Separate analyses with the Chevy Chase sample alone also showed no significant improvement for active versus sham FNS treatment (p > .22).

Tender Points. According to the criteria of Simms et al. (1988) a tender point score reduction of at least 25% or a tender point score of 14 or less (1991) is a clinically meaningful treatment response. As Table 3 shows, no more than 25% of those in either treatment group met either of the Simms et al. response criteria at session 22 or one-week post-treatment. The percentages did not differ significantly between treatment groups.

Symptom Scales. Table 4 shows the baseline and endpoint symptom scale scores. GEE analyses showed no significant treatment-by-time interactions, indicating that symptom reports did not differ between the FNS and sham groups over the course of treatment on any of the seven scales. Analyses were repeated using data from sessions 5, 13, and 19 only, when participants remained on their concomitant medications, to eliminate the "cold-turkey withdrawal effect" associated with their discontinuance for 48 hours preceding EEG mapping (sessions 9, 16, and 22). These results were not substantively different.

TABLE 3. Summary of Treatment Outcomes by Time Point and Treatment Group–Primary Pain Measures Baseline and End Point Scores[a]

	Pretreatment		Session 22		Post-Treatment		P Value[b]	
	FNS	Sham	FNS	Sham	FNS	Sham	Session 22	Post-Treatment
	(n = 31)	(n = 28)	(n = 31)	(n = 28)	(n = 31)	(n = 28)		
Dolorimetry, mean kg/1.54 cm^2 (sd)	1.47 (0.96)	1.72 (0.81)	1.67 (1.09)[c]	1.56 (0.97)	1.47 (0.96)[c]	1.45 (1.01)	.11	.22
Tender points responders, n (%)			7 (22.6)[d]	7 (25.0)	4 (12.9)[d]	5 (17.9)	1.0	.72

[a] Mean (sd) scores for FNS group at session 22 and 1-week post-treatment include last observation carried forward score for one subject.

[b] FNS, Flexyx Neurotherapy System®; P values for dolorimetry are for the treatment-by-session interaction in the general estimating equation (GEE) models. Dolorimetry score statistics are based on modeling the measures at sessions 9, 16, 22 and 1-week post-treatment follow-up as a linear function of baseline score, treatment, site, session, treatment by session, and site by session (site-by-treatment and treatment-by-site-by-session terms were non-significant and dropped from the models). P values for tender point responders are based on Fisher's exact test.

[c] Mean (sd) includes last observation score for one subject who dropped out before session 22 and post-treatment evaluations but was included in GEE analysis.

[d] Includes session 9 score carried forward for one subject who dropped out before session 22 and post-treatment evaluations.

TABLE 4. Summary of Treatment Outcomes by Time Point and Treatment Group–Specific Symptom Severity Scales Baseline and End Point Scores

	Pretreatment		Session 22		Post-Treatment		P Value[b]	
	FNS	Sham	FNS	Sham	FNS	Sham	Session 22	Post-Treatment
	(n = 31)	(n = 28)	(n = 31)	(n = 28)	(n = 31)	(n = 28)		
Generalized pain, mean (sd)	6.68 (1.45)	5.96 (2.01)	5.03 (2.30)	5.07 (2.36)	5.33 (2.58)	5.29 (2.26)	.30	.33
Specific pain, mean (sd)	7.35 (1.50)	7.18 (1.61)	6.23 (2.28)	6.00 (2.24)	6.17 (2.38)	6.04 (2.12)	.60	.61
Short-term memory mean (sd)	5.19 (1.76)	5.21 (2.22)	4.40 (2.04)	4.64 (2.09)	4.40 (2.13)	4.54 (2.08)	.53	.38[b]
Concentration, mean (sd)	5.39 (1.56)	5.25 (2.27)	4.47 (2.05)	4.61 (2.20)	4.70 (2.48)	4.61 (2.28)	.88	.92
Multitasking, mean (sd)	4.71 (2.37)	5.39 (2.18)	3.87 (2.27)	4.46 (2.24)	4.20 (2.75)	4.29 (2.11)	.67	.82
Depression, mean (sd)	4.29 (2.21)	4.14 (2.32)	3.43 (2.61)	3.11 (2.02)	3.83 (3.07)	3.71 (2.39)	.88	.76
Fatigue, mean (sd)	7.19 (2.10)	6.11 (2.30)	5.83 (2.36)	5.57 (2.32)	6.23 (2.60)	5.61 (2.27)	.40	.49

[a] FNS, Flexyx Neurotherapy System®; P values are for the treatment-by-session interaction in the general estimating equation (GEE) models. Statistics are based on modeling the scores at sessions 5, 9, 13, 16, 19, and 22 and at 1-week post-treatment follow-up as a linear function of pretreatment baseline (session 1) scores, and treatment, site, session, and treatment-by-session (site by session, site-by-treatment, and treatment-by-site-by-session terms were non-significant and dropped from the models, except as noted in footnote b). For each symptom, severity range = 1 (none) to 10 (extremely severe). One subject in FNS group dropped out after session 13 but was included in the GEE analysis for both session 22 and 1-week post-treatment outcomes.

[b] Separate analysis was conducted with the Chevy Chase sample because the site-by-treatment interaction was significant (p < .05) at 1-week post-treatment; the treatment-by-session interaction was not significant in this site-specific analysis.

CNS Dysfunction Questionnaire. We were particularly interested in change in cognitive complaints, especially "fibro-fog," characterized by "foggy" thinking, reduced ability to focus attention and maintain concentration, and forgetfulness (Mueller et al., 2001). On this self-report symptom measure, there was no statistically significant treatment-by-time in-

teraction for the total score or on any of the instrument's eight subscales. Treatment-by-site differences were found on the sensory (p < .01) and movement (p < .04) subscales but separate analyses with the Chevy Chase sample revealed no significant difference in outcomes between active and sham FNS.

Symptom Checklist-90-R. This instrument

was administered at pre-treatment screening and post-treatment follow-up. As shown in Table 5, there were no significant differential treatment effects on any of the three global distress change scores. On all global scores and the nine symptom scales (data not shown), Chicago participants had higher mean scores both pre- and post-treatment. Moreover, except for the paranoid ideation scale, mean scores were higher in the active treatment group compared with the sham treatment group. Re-analysis limited to the Chevy Chase sample (N = 49) showed no significant pre-post treatment difference between active and sham FNS groups.

Fibromyalgia Impact Questionnaire. Table 6 shows that there were no significant treatment effects for any FIQ item. For the "depressed" and "number of symptoms" items, data were reanalyzed with the Chevy Chase sample alone because there was a significant site-by-treatment group interaction. The treatment-by-time interaction was not significant for either item, indicating no significant difference between the two treatment groups.

EEG Maps and Treatment Response. As shown in Table 7, the active and sham FNS groups did not differ significantly in EEG amplitude change (means and standard deviations) from pre-treatment to the final treatment session. The only EEG correlate of global improvement scales outcome was alpha mean amplitude, which decreased significantly in

sham-treated PGI-I responders compared with the sham-treated nonresponders (b = 1.19; Wald test = 3.83, df = 1, p = .05). There was a trend for the alpha standard deviation to be related to PGI-I response in the active FNS group (b = −3.51; Wald test = 3.24, df = 1, p = .07). Delta mean and standard deviation and total EEG amplitude mean and standard deviation were not related to CGI-I or PGI-I response in treatment group- and site-adjusted logistic regression analyses.

A pre-treatment delta/alpha EEG amplitude ratio > 1 was related to PGI-I but not CGI-I response ratings. This relationship was significant at one-week post-treatment; participants with delta/alpha > 1, compared with those who had a ratio < 1, had more than a six-fold higher odds (odds ratio = 6.44, 95% confidence interval = 1.65-25.17; p = .007) of PGI-I-rated "remission." This relationship did not differ by treatment group; the ratio-by-treatment interaction was not significant. At session 22, there was only a trend for the delta/alpha ratio to be related to response (b = 1.12; Wald test = 3.27, df = 1, p = .07).

Adequacy of the Blinding–Participants' Guess of Treatment Group Assignment

Before unblinding at the one-week post-treatment assessment, participants were asked what treatment they thought they had received. Those in both treatment groups were equally accurate in "guessing" their treatment. Twenty (67%; n = 30) in the active FNS group and 19 (68%; n = 28) in the sham FNS group correctly identified the treatment they had received (Fisher's exact test, p [2-tailed] = 1.0). According to the binomial test, neither proportion was significantly greater than chance (50%) expectation (active FNS, p = .10; sham, p = .09). There was no significant site difference in guessing correctly (Chicago, 60%; Chevy Chase, 68%; Fisher's exact test, p [2-tailed] = 1.0).

Safety and Side Effects

Of the 59 participants who completed at least one post-randomization assessment, 31 (52.5%) reported at least one side effect at any time during treatment. Two additional participants, one

TABLE 5. Symptom Checklist (SCL)-90-R Global Indices of Psychological Distress Scores[a]

	Pretreatment		Post-Treatment		
	FNS	Sham	FNS	Sham	P Value[b]
	(n = 30)	(n = 27)	(n = 30)	(n = 27)	
GSI, mean (sd)	0.75 (0.48)	0.61 (0.34)	0.65 (0.54)	0.54 (0.44)	.87
PST, mean (sd)	37.4 (18.3)	30.7 (12.0)	32.7 (16.4)	29.7 (16.1)	.67
PSDI, mean (sd)	1.73 (0.37)	1.72 (0.37)	1.63 (0.44)	1.59 (0.41)	.25

[a] FNS, Flexyx Neurotherapy System®; GSI, Global Severity Index; PST, Positive Symptom Total; PSDI, Positive Symptom Distress Index. N = 57, pretreatment SCL-90-R not completed by one sham-treated subject and one-week post-treatment SCL-90-R not completed by one FNS-treated subject who terminated before the final session.

[b] P value for treatment-by-session interaction, representing differential improvement for active versus sham FNS treatment. Repeated measures analysis of covariance model includes treatment group, site, and all interactions.

TABLE 6. Fibromyalgia Impact Questionnaire Indices[a]

	Pretreatment		Post-Treatment		
	FNS	Sham	FNS	Sham	P Value[b]
	(n = 30)	(n = 28)	(n = 30)	(n = 28)	
Physical functioning, mean, (sd)	1.41 (0.77)	1.32 (0.85)	1.28 (0.82)	1.15 (0.87)	.34
# days feeling good,[c] mean (sd)	1.43 (2.10)	1.61 (1.85)	2.57 (2.60)	2.50 (2.27)	.92
# days slept well,[c] mean (sd)	1.77 (2.14)	1.82 (1.93)	2.43 (2.28)	2.57 (2.39)	.61
# days missed work,[c,d] mean, (sd)	0.55 (1.39)	0.22 (0.73)	0.55 (1.54)	0.08 (0.35)	.46
Pain/symptoms interfere with work,[d] mean, (sd)	4.30 (2.98)	4.39 (2.73)	3.00 (2.79)	3.39 (3.11)	.16
Pain severity, mean (sd)	6.27 (2.41)	6.43 (1.79)	5.23 (2.34)	5.57 (2.23)	.33
Tiredness, mean (sd)	7.63 (1.50)	6.75 (1.58)	6.40 (2.30)	5.61 (2.13)	.81
Waking tired, mean (sd)	8.00 (1.44)	6.75 (1.80)	6.43 (2.18)	5.57 (2.57)	.12
Stiffness, mean (sd)	6.97 (2.17)	6.43 (2.08)	5.47 (2.83)	5.43 (2.17)	.24
Tense/anxious, mean (sd)	5.30 (2.88)	5.04 (2.55)	4.77 (2.79)	3.82 (2.63)	.95
Depressed, mean (sd)	3.23 (1.94)	3.82 (2.42)	3.63 (3.03)	3.39 (2.77)	.17
# symptoms,[e] mean (sd)	17.53 (4.55)	15.68 (4.18)	14.87 (5.76)	13.79 (5.26)	.70

[a] N = 58, one-week post-treatment questionnaire not completed by one FNS-treated subject who terminated before the final session. FNS, Flexyx Neurotherapy System®.

[b] P value for treatment-by-session interaction, representing differential improvement for active versus sham FNS treatment. Repeated measures analysis of covariance model includes treatment group, site, and all interactions.

[c] Number (#) of days in past week (0-7).

[d] Based on 38 subjects employed at study intake, 20 in the active FNS group and 18 in the sham FNS group. Sites combined because only 3 Chicago subjects were employed.

[e] Number (#) of symptoms (0-29).

TABLE 7. FNS EEG Maps[a]

	Pretreatment		Session 22		
	FNS	Sham	FNS	Sham	P Value[b]
	(n = 30)	(n = 28)	(n = 30)	(n = 28)	
Alpha[c] mean (sd)	4.07 (1.27)	4.47 (1.96)	4.20 (1.78)	4.62 (2.25)	.86
Alpha[c] SD, mean (sd)	1.03 (0.38)	1.05 (0.49)	1.03 (0.45)	1.15 (0.63)	.75
Delta[d] mean (sd)	3.69 (0.55)	3.86 (0.77)	3.76 (0.84)	4.04 (1.14)	.76
Delta[d] SD, mean (sd)	1.20 (0.22)	1.41 (0.55)	1.18 (0.33)	1.33 (0.38)	.90
Total, mean (sd)	7.80 (1.34)	8.52 (1.93)	7.94 (1.99)	8.63 (2.42)	.87
Total SD, mean (sd)	1.42 (0.34)	1.61 (0.58)	1.35 (0.42)	1.54 (0.42)	.62

[a] FNS, Flexyx Neurotherapy System®. Pretreatment versus session 22 recordings of EEG amplitude averaged across 21 scalp sites, means (microvolts) and standard deviations (SD). N = 58, post-treatment recording not available for one FNS-treated subject who terminated before the final session.

[b] P value for treatment group-by-session interaction, representing differential improvement for active versus sham FNS treatment. Model includes treatment group, site, and all interactions.

[c] Alpha = 8-12 Hz.

[d] Delta = 1-4 Hz.

in the active FNS group and one in the sham FNS group, reported a side effect only at the one-week follow-up. The percentages reporting side effects differed significantly ($\chi^2 = 7.35$, df = 1, p < .007) between active (74.2%) and sham (35.7%) treatment groups. The symptom reported most commonly, fatigue/tiredness, was reported by 13 participants (10 in the active FNS group). Pain, including headache, was reported by 10 participants (6 in the active FNS group). Three participants in the active FNS group reported pain/fatigue associated with stopping their medications at the FNS mapping sessions (sessions 9, 16, and 22). Four participants in the active FNS group reported sleep, drowsiness, or change in sleep patterns. Three participants in the active FNS group reported stiffness or muscle spasms. No other symptom was reported by more than two participants. Most side effects occurred early in the course of treatment; 21 participants (15 with FNS, 6 with sham) reported at least one at session 5, diminishing to only 10 (6 with FNS, 2 with sham) by the last two sessions and 8 at follow-up. Earlier in treatment, most side effects did not affect functioning. During later sessions, 50%-64% of side effects were rated as severe enough to interfere with functioning. For two participants receiving active FNS, side effects were rated as "nullifies therapeutic effect"; one participant did not report this level of severity until the one-week post-treatment assessment. None dropped out due to side effects, but in a few cases treatment sessions were suspended temporarily before resuming.

DISCUSSION

The major finding in this first randomized controlled clinical trial of FNS for treating FMS was that only the clinician-rated global impressions scores detected a treatment-related response, which persisted through one-week post-treatment follow-up only for the combined partial and full responders. Significantly more participants treated with active compared with sham FNS were rated as partially or fully remitted. This result is tempered by the finding that CGI-I and PGI-I outcomes were discrepant, with clinicians' ratings more optimistic than those of participants. Moreover, a pre-treatment delta/alpha EEG amplitude ratio > 1 was associated with PGI-I (but not CGI-I) response independent of treatment group assignment.

Improvement in global symptoms has been used to measure outcome in clinical trials involving other somatic conditions, such as irritable bowel syndrome (Brandt et al., 2002). As in irritable bowel syndrome, the clinician's treatment strategy for managing FNS is symptom-driven, so we also examined symptom outcomes. Dolorimetry ratings and tender point counts did not improve significantly more in the active than in the sham FNS group, and other symptom, psychological, and functioning measures showed no benefit for active FNS compared with sham.

Three studies on the efficacy of FNS have been published and two, both by the same group, involved patients with fibromyalgia. The first was a retrospective study of 252 patients referred with fibromyalgia, but only 157 met ACR criteria plus had sleep and mental processing problems (Donaldson, Sella & Mueller, 1998). Only 44 completed treatment and 40 reported symptomatic improvement (6 had no symptoms). EEG neurofeedback was combined with sEMG biofeedback and other myofascial treatment, and continued until symptoms reached a plateau, usually after three to six months of the integrated regimen.

The second study, described earlier (Mueller et al., 2001), involved 30 consecutive outpatients with ACR-diagnosed fibromyalgia (5 also had chronic fatigue syndrome). There was no control group, treatment was non-blinded clinical practice, and patients paid for treatment. All but four had at least one additional non-pharmacological therapeutic modality (sEMG, physical and/or massage therapy) and continued treatment until they experienced sufficient symptomatic relief, or ran out of time or money for further therapy. Their patients averaged 51.9 hours of treatment over 14.7 weeks, compared with 22 sessions over a minimum of 11 weeks in our study.

Did we under-treat? Mueller et al. (2001) reported that pain measures (percent of body involved in pain, pressure algometry, tender points; only 17 of 30 had the latter two reassessments) as well as other fibromyalgia symptoms improved significantly at the conclusion of active treatment. Follow-up assessment indicated that, compared to pre-treatment, patients indicated they were on average $62.2 \pm 21.6\%$ improved 3 to 18 months (mean = 8.2 months) post-treatment.

In the third study (Schoenberger et al., 2001), 12 patients with traumatic brain injury were randomized to receive 25 FNS treatment sessions over 5 to 8 weeks immediately or after a delay of 6 to 8 weeks ("wait-list" control group). The immediate active treatment group was compared at time 2 with the delayed (control) group, which was post-treatment for the former group and pre-treatment for the latter group. The active treatment group improved significantly on a range of symptoms. Particularly relevant for fibromyalgia vis-à-vis the "fibro-fog" symptoms (which we measured with the CNS Dysfunction Questionnaire and the concentration, short-term memory, and multitasking symptom scales), significant improvement was observed on measures of cognitive functioning.

Based on the promising results of these three studies, we conducted this double-blind, placebo-controlled clinical trial. The results raise questions regarding FNS's treatment efficacy as well as study validity. What happened?

Does FNS really work or did the global impressions scale measure some other aspect of improvement, such as the quality of the participants' relationship with the therapist? The CGI-I, not the PGI-I, rating was the a priori primary outcome and the outcome on which the power analysis was based. In fact, CGI-I active vs. sham response differences were 23% and 19% at session 22 and one-week post-treatment, respectively. Including partial responders in the analysis of therapeutic effect, the differences were 31.7% at session 22 and 25% at one-week post-treatment. These latter differences are close to our predicted 30% difference, the basis for our power analysis.

Nevertheless, how can we explain the discrepancy between clinician and participant global impressions ratings? For example, did therapists "break the blind" and were ratings biased according to expectations and awareness of treatment allocation (note, we had no measure of clinicians' "guesses," only participants' guesses)? Was site heterogeneity, either in type of FMS patients seen, the therapists/evaluators, or treatment orientation at these two different geographically distinct locales a source of study invalidity? Was the sham treatment a true placebo (i.e., was it really inactive biologically)? Are 22 sessions an adequate treatment regimen? Was the experimental design inconsistent with actual FNS use in clinical practice in regards to the number of treatment sessions and concomitant interventions?

Did the blind remain intact? Although active- and sham-treated participants were equally accurate in guessing treatment assignment, those in the active group were more likely to rate the study treatment as more effective than previous treatment and those in the sham group were more likely to rate study treatment as no different or worse than previous treatment. Moreover, of those rating themselves as remitted, FNS treatment was rated as more effective than previous treatments by 100% at session 22 and 93% at one-week post-treatment. Of those who did not rate themselves as remitted, only 29% at session 22 and 33% at one-week post-treatment rated the treatment as more effective than previous treatment. Thus, there is some evidence that treatment "guesses," perceived comparative treatment efficacy and, to a lesser extent, self-rated improvement (PGI-I) were associated.

An important methodological issue must be raised here–does the site heterogeneity represent true difference in FMS patients, particularly in regards to symptom severity, or does it indicate a lack of inter-rater reliability? Therapists received the same training in administering treatment and recording EEG activity (FNS maps). However, dolorimetry raters did not undergo inter-rater reliability training. Chicago raters were two masters-level trained rheumatology nurse-practitioners with considerable experience in conducting dolorimetry examinations. In Chevy Chase, four people with diverse clinical backgrounds did the dolorimetry ratings–a registered nurse, two myofascial/nationally certified massage therapists, and a very experienced sEMG therapist. Two of these raters left the study but trained their replacements. Dolorimetry has been considered more objective than tender point examination; nevertheless, discrepancies between dolorimetry and tender point digital exam have been reported (Cott et al., 1992; Wolfe, Ross, Anderson, & Russell, 1995; Wolfe et al., 1990). This is a moot point in our case because tender point counts were derived from dolorimetry as described by Mueller et al. (2001); independent digital examination was not done.

Excepting the therapist CGI, all other outcome instruments are participant-rated. Although no specific inter-rater reliability training on the CGI-I scale was conducted, there also were no statistically significant site differences on this outcome. Analytically, concerns can be raised regarding the comparatively smaller Chicago sample. To compensate, site was included as a factor and separate site-specific analyses were conducted when significant interactions involving site were found. Another problem was that the study's power was diminished after the third site was dropped midway through the study, which was compounded by an effect size that was smaller than expected.

While the pathogenesis of fibromyalgia is not well understood, the proposed theories share the postulate that these patients do not perceive or respond normally to physical or psychological stresses (Block, 1999). These stresses are likely to be multifactorial, requiring a combined therapeutic approach. Furthermore, not all fibromyalgia may be alike– fibromyalgia attributed to different etiologic factors may respond differently in terms of rate and completeness. For example, FMS acquired post-infection (9% of our sample) may be slower to respond compared with FMS that developed post-physical trauma (39% of our sample); 13% of our sample reported both of these factors and 39% reported "other/unknown" precipitants. Donaldson, Sella, and Mueller (1998) reported that those who responded only slightly gave histories of fibromyalgia triggered by a viral infection whereas those who were greatly improved or symptom-free gave histories of an antecedent trauma.

A possible limitation of our study is that those with debilitating chronic fatigue were not included. Thus, our sample may have been somewhat atypical of FMS patients seeking treatment. In fact, our sample could have included patients with co-existing chronic fatigue symptoms but they were not the more severe cases.

The most important finding may be that for fibromyalgia patients EEG treatment alone is not sufficient for recovery. In this study we examined the therapeutic efficacy of FNS monotherapy. Clinically, fibromyalgia patients treated with FNS receive a multimodal treatment regimen including the sEMG and myofascial treatment as well, because the pain from the body tends to perpetuate the CNS problems, preventing recovery (Donaldson, Nelson & Schulz, 1998; Mueller et al., 2001). It may be necessary to combine the EEG stimulation with sEMG to get rid of muscle imbalances that cause spasms. sEMG is used to teach people to retrain their muscles, thereby reducing muscle spasm. The EMG identifies the problem, and the patient is given specific exercises to do at home. The sEMG treatment is coordinated with myofascial release treatment. The fascial constrictions that build up over years of imbalances have to be removed by myofascial therapy in order for the patient to regain full muscle function. The EEG stimulation may facilitate muscle relaxation as well as softening of trigger points/tender points by some as yet not understood mechanism. Lichtbroun, Raicer, and Smith (2001) noted similarly that cranial electrotherapy stimulation, while more effective than a sham treatment comparator for treating fibromyalgia, has potentiated the effects of biofeedback when the two were given together for migraine (Brotman, 1989). Interactions among these various modalities and the need to individualize treatments complicate the design and conduct of clinical trials involving FNS or other EEG-based stimulation for fibromyalgia.

Finally, Paterson and Dieppe (2005) noted that placebo or sham controlled trial designs used for evaluating complex non-pharmaceutical interventions may generate false negative results. Reduced active–sham treatment effect sizes and inadequately powered studies can result from failure to consider that factors such as empathy and focused attention may be integral, not "non-specific," aspects of the total treatment effect. This certainly is a consideration in FNS therapy.

Continued investigation of non-pharmacological interventions in well-designed controlled clinical trials is essential. Wallace (1997), citing Pioro-Boisset, Esdaile, and Fitzcharles (1996), noted that in Canada 91% of FMS patients, compared with 63% of control rheumatic disease patients, use complementary and alternative medicine measures. Our negative study may have been due at least in part to an experimental design that was inconsistent with how FNS is used in clinical practice, such as in terms of concomitant interventions and number of treatment sessions. Thus, differences between research and clinical practice settings in how and when FNS is administered may account for discrepant treatment outcomes.

REFERENCES

Block, S. R. (1999). On the nature of rheumatism. *Arthritis Care and Research, 12*, 129-138.

Brandt, L. J., Bjorkman, D., Fennerty, M. B., Locke, G. R., Olden, K., Peterson, W., et al. (2002). Systematic review on the management of irritable bowel syndrome in North America. *American Journal of Gastroenterology, 97* (11 Suppl.), S7-26.

Brotman, P. (1989). Transcranial electrotherapy: Low-intensity transcranial electrostimulation improves the efficacy of thermal biofeedback and quieting reflex training in the treatment of classical migraine headache. *American Journal of Electromedicine, 6*, 120-123.

Budzynski, T. H. (1999). From EEG to neurofeedback. In J.R. Evans & A. Abarbanel (Eds.), *Introduction to quantitative EEG and neurofeedback* (pp. 65-79). San Diego, CA: Academic Press.

Burckhardt, C. S., Clark, S. R., & Bennett, R. M. (1991). The Fibromyalgia Impact Questionnaire: Development and validation. *Journal of Rheumatology, 18*, 728-733.

Burckhardt, C. S., Clark, S. R., & Bennett, R. M. (1993). Fibromyalgia and quality of life: A comparative analysis. *Journal of Rheumatology, 20*, 475-479.

Callahan, L. F., & Blalock, S. J., (1997). Behavioral and social research in rheumatology. *Current Opinion in Rheumatology, 9*, 126-132.

Cott, A., Parkinson, W., Bell, M. J., Adachi, J., Bedard, M., Cividino, A., et al. (1992). Interrater reliability of the tender point criterion for fibromyalgia. *Journal of Rheumatology, 19*, 1955-1959.

Derogatis, L. R. (1994). SCL-90-R® (Symptom Checklist-90-R). *Administration, scoring, and procedures manual* (3rd ed.). Minneapolis, MN: National Computer Systems, Inc.

Diggle, P.J., Heagerty, P. J., Liang, K.Y., & Zeger, S. L. (2002). *Analysis of longitudinal data* (2nd ed.). New York, NY: Oxford University Press.

Donaldson, C. C. S., Nelson, D. V., & Schulz, R. (1998). Disinhibition in the gamma motoneuron circuitry: A neglected mechanism for understanding myofascial pain syndromes. *Applied Psychophysiology & Biofeedback, 23*, 43-58.

Donaldson, C. C. S., Sella, G. E., & Mueller, H. H. (1998). Fibromyalgia. A retrospective study of 252 consecutive referrals. *Canadian Journal of Clinical Medicine, 5*, 116-121,124-127.

Flor, H., Birbaumer, N., & Turk, D. C. (1990). The psychobiology of chronic pain. *Advances in Behaviour Research and Therapy, 12*, 47-84.

Forseth, K. O., Gran, J. T., Husby, G., & Forre, O. (1999). Prognostic factors for the development of fibromyalgia in women with self-reported musculoskeletal pain. A prospective study. *Journal of Rheumatology, 26*, 2458-2467.

Guy, W. (1976). ECDEU *Assessment manual for psychopharmacology–Revised* (DHEW Pub No. ADM 76-338) (pp. 218-222). Rockville, MD: U.S. Department of Health, Education, and Welfare, Public Health Service, Alcohol, Drug Abuse, and Mental Health Administration, NIMH Psychopharmacology Research Branch, Division of Extramural Research Programs.

Hosmer, D. W., & Lemeshow, S. (2000). *Applied logistic regression* (2nd ed.). New York: John Wiley & Sons, Inc.

Laibow, R. (1999). Medical applications of neurobiofeedback. In J.R. Evans & A. Abarbanel (Eds). *Introduction to quantitative EEG and neurofeedback* (pp. 83-102). San Diego, CA: Academic Press.

Lawrence, R. C., Helmick, C. G., Arnett, F. C., Deyo, R. A., Felson, D.T., Giannini, E. H., et al. (1998). Estimates of the prevalence of arthritis and selected musculoskeletal disorders in the United States. *Arthritis and Rheumatism, 41*, 778-799.

Lichtbroun, A. S., Raicer, M.-M. C., Smith, R. B. (2001). The treatment of fibromyalgia with cranial electrotherapy stimulation. *Journal of Clinical Rheumatology, 7*, 72-78.

Makela, M. O. (1999). Is fibromyalgia a distinct clinical entity? The epidemiologist's evidence. *Bailliere's Clinical Rheumatology, 13*, 415-419.

McBeth, J., Macfarlane, G. J., Hunt, I. M., & Silman, A. J. (2001). Risk factors for persistent chronic widespread pain: A community based study. *Rheumatology, 40*, 95-101.

Mueller, H. H., Donaldson, C. C. S., Nelson, D. V., & Lyman, M. (2001). Treatment of fibromyalgia incorporating EEG-driven stimulation: A clinical outcomes study. *Journal of Clinical Psychology, 57*, 933-952.

Ochs, L. (1993). New lights on lights, sound, and the brain. *Megabrain Report: Journal of Mind Technology, 2*, 48-52.

Ochs, L. (1997). *EDS: Background and operation. EEG-driven pico-photic stimulation.* Walnut Creek, CA: Flexyx LLC.

Paterson, C., & Dieppe, P. (2005). Characteristic and incidental (placebo) effects in complex interventions such as acupuncture. *British Medical Journal, 330*, 1202-1205.

Pioro-Boisset, M., Esdaile, J. M., & Fitzcharles, M.-A. (1996). Alternative medicine use in fibromyalgia syndrome. *Arthritis Care and Research, 9*, 13-17.

Rossy, L. A., Buckelew, S. P., Dorr, N., Hagglund, K .J., Thayer, J. F., McIntosh, M. J., et al. (1999). A meta-analysis of fibromyalgia treatment interventions. *Annals of Behavioral Medicine, 21*, 180-191.

Rothman, K. J. (1990). No adjustments are needed for multiple comparisons. *Epidemiology, 1*, 43-46.

Scharf, M. B. (2003, June). The effects of sodium oxybate on clinical symptoms and sleep patterns in fibromyalgia. Paper presented at the 17th annual meeting of the Associated Professional Sleep Societies, Chicago, IL.

Schoenberger, N. E., Shiflett, S. C., Esty, M. L., Ochs, L., & Matheis, R. J. (2001). Flexyx Neurotherapy System in the treatment of traumatic brain injury: An initial evaluation. *Journal of Head Trauma Rehabilitation, 16* (3), 260-274.

Schwartz M. S. (1995). Fibromyalgia syndrome. In M.S. Schwartz (Ed.), *Biofeedback: A practitioner's guide* (2nd ed., pp. 803-819). New York: Guilford Press.

Simms, R. W. (1994). Controlled trials of therapy in fibromyalgia syndrome. *Balliere's Clinical Rheumatology, 8,* 917-934.

Simms, R. W., Felson, D. T., & Goldenberg, D. L. (1988). Criteria for response to treatment in fibromyalgia. [Abstract]. *Arthritis and Rheumatism, 31* (Suppl.), S100.

Simms, R. W., Felson, D. T., & Goldenberg, D. L. (1991). Development of preliminary criteria for response to treatment in fibromyalgia syndrome. *Journal of Rheumatology, 18,* 1558-1563.

Simms, R. W., Goldenberg, D. L., Felson, D. T., & Mason, J. H. (1988). Tenderness in 75 anatomic sites: Distinguishing fibromyalgia patients from controls. *Arthritis and Rheumatism, 31,* 182-187.

Staud, R. (2002). Evidence of involvement of central neural mechanisms in generating fibromyalgia pain. *Current Rheumatology Reports, 4,* 299-305.

Tunks, E., Crook, J., Norman, G., & Kalaher, S. (1988). Tender points in fibromyalgia. *Pain, 34,* 11-19.

Wallace, D. J. (1997). The fibromyalgia syndrome. *Annals of Medicine, 29,* 9-21.

White, K. P., & Harth, M. (1996). An analytical review of 24 controlled clinical trials for fibromyalgia syndrome (FMS). *Pain, 64,* 211-219.

White, K. P., & Harth, M. (1999). The occurrence and impact of generalized pain. *Bailliere's Clinical Rheumatology, 13,* 379-389.

White, K. P., Speechley, M., Harth, M., & Ostbye, T. (1999). The London Fibromyalgia Epidemiology Study: Direct health care costs of fibromyalgia syndrome in London, Canada. *Journal of Rheumatology, 26,* 885-889.

Wolfe, F. and the Vancouver Fibromyalgia Consensus Group. (1996). The fibromyalgia syndrome: A consensus report on fibromyalgia and disability. *Journal of Rheumatology, 23,* 534-539.

Wolfe, F., & Cathey, M. A. (1985). The epidemiology of tender points: A prospective study of 1520 patients. *Journal of Rheumatology, 12,* 1164-1168.

Wolfe, F., Ross, K., Anderson, J., & Russell, I. J. (1995). Aspects of fibromyalgia in the general population: Sex, pain threshold, and fibromyalgia symptoms. *Journal of Rheumatology, 22,* 151-156.

Wolfe, F., Ross, K., Anderson, J., Russell, I. J., & Hebert, L. (1995). The prevalence and characteristics of fibromyalgia in the general population. *Arthritis and Rheumatism, 38,* 19-28.

Wolfe, F., Smythe, H. A., Yunus, M. B., Bennett, R. M., Bombardier, C., Goldenberg, D. L., et al. (1990). The American College of Rheumatology 1990 criteria for the classification of fibromyalgia. Report of the Multicenter Criteria Committee. *Arthritis and Rheumatism, 33,* 160-172.

doi:10.1300/J184v10n02_03

Comment on the Treatment of Fibromyalgia Syndrome Using Low-Intensity Neurofeedback with the Flexyx Neurotherapy System: A Randomized Controlled Clinical Trial, or How to Go Crazy Over Nearly Nothing

Len Ochs, PhD

SUMMARY. This commentary to the Kravitz, Esty, Katz, and Fawcett (2006) study reports a significant flaw in the hardware used in the study. This hardware problem was not known at the time of the study and was only revealed later in technical analyses of the equipment. The difference in outcome between the Kravitz et al. study versus other studies using low energy electromagnetic feedback stimulation may be explained by this analysis. doi:10.1300/J184v10n02_04 *[Article copies available for a fee from The Haworth Document Delivery Service: 1-800-HAWORTH. E-mail address: <docdelivery@haworthpress.com> Website: <http://www.HaworthPress.com> © 2006 by The Haworth Press, Inc. All rights reserved.]*

KEYWORDS. Neurotherapy, Flexyx Neurotherapy System, fibromyalgia, controlled clinical trial, treatment, neurofeedback

An element missing in the Kravitz, Esty, Katz and Fawcett (2006) study is a discussion of the equipment used in formal and informal studies preceding that study, as well as in the Kravitz study, from the perspective of the underlying mechanism of the properties of the carrier medium that was used for the feedback stimulation. The Kravitz report treats all versions of the neurofeedback that were used as one undifferentiated type. Furthermore, there was no discussion of electromagnetic characteristics of the different EEG preamplifiers. In fact, from what we now know, it is probable that the configuration of the I-330 C2 accounts for both the negative results and the side effects seen in the current study. The stimulation characteristics, electromagnetic characteristics or light of equipment used in previous studies are shown in Table 1.

First, a word about the lights embedded in the glasses that were worn for light feedback in the past and in the Kravitz et al. study. Long experience with the older I-400 preamplifier systems had led us to exclusively use lights that were

Len Ochs is affiliated with Ochs Labs, Sebastopol, CA.

Address correspondence to: Len Ochs, 8151 Elphick Lane, Sebastopol, CA 94596 (E-mail: lochs@earthlink.net).

[Haworth co-indexing entry note]: "Comment on the Treatment of Fibromyalgia Syndrome Using Low-Intensity Neurofeedback with the Flexyx Neurotherapy System: A Randomized Controlled Clinical Trial, or How to Go Crazy Over Nearly Nothing." Ochs, Len. Co-published simultaneously in *Journal of Neurotherapy* (The Haworth Medical Press, an imprint of The Haworth Press, Inc.) Vol. 10, No. 2/3, 2006, pp. 59-61; and: *LENS: The Low Energy Neurofeedback System* (ed: D. Corydon Hammond) The Haworth Medical Press, an imprint of The Haworth Press, Inc., 2006, pp. 59-61. Single or multiple copies of this article are available for a fee from The Haworth Document Delivery Service [1-800-HAWORTH, 9:00 a.m. - 5:00 p.m. (EST). E-mail address: docdelivery@haworthpress.com].

Available online at http://jn.haworthpress.com
© 2006 by The Haworth Press, Inc. All rights reserved.
doi:10.1300/J184v10n02_04

TABLE 1. Comparison of Electromagnetic Fields in Equipment in Previous Studies.

Author	EEG Model	EM-characteristics	Feedback Carrier	Observations
Schoenberger et al.	I-400	None	Light	Positive outcome
Mueller et al.	I-400	None	Light	Positive outcome
Donaldson et al.	I-400	None	Light	Positive outcome
Kravitz et al.	I-330 C2	Strong	EMF+Light	Negative

taped over with up to 60 layers of black vinyl electrical tape. In fact, at times the layers of tape were so thick that they pressed upon the eyes of the patients wearing the glasses. Some of the therapists joked about the possibility that one or two photons per week might pass through the tape to the eyes. No light was ever visible under this condition, even though the results of the supposed visual feedback seemed satisfactory.

When the new I-330 C2 preamplifier was introduced, however, the strength of the stimulation seemed to be much greater than from the previous I-400. J&J Engineering worked with us to reduce current flow to the lights until any further reduction in light intensity would reduce the coded feedback information to a level lower than the thermal noise of the electrons passing through the wire to the lights in the glasses.

Because one fibromyalgia patient fell asleep for at least 45 minutes after each I-330 C2 session, I was asked to assess the problem and to see if I could further reduce the intensity of the feedback. At the start of the session I removed the glasses from the patient and moved them as far away from her face as the cable from the I-330 C2 would allow me–approximately four feet. I pressed a graphic button on the screen four times as I pulled the glasses further and further away, delivering what I thought was four seconds of feedback from the lights in the glasses. Each time I pressed the button I could see her EEG respond to the feedback impulse. For the first time since this patient began using the system, she was energized enough that she was able to take a reasonably long walk after the session, and she was both free from fibromyalgia pain and from mental fog. As we will see, what really happened is that there was one less

cable–the cable to the glasses–draped over the patient.

Early clinical use of the I-330 C2 EEG showed the same kinds of untoward effects as reported in the study. The presence of these effects impelled us to reduce the strength of the radio frequencies. Radio frequency interference filters were used to reduce the intensity of the electromagnetic field. This field was conducted by the EEG leads down to the patient's head. This made the EEG leads bidirectional conductors, carrying the EEG signal to the EEG preamplifier in one direction, and the electromagnetic field with the feedback signal, to the head in the other direction.

Again, the therapists using what was then called the Flexyx Neurofeedback System (FNS) system joked that I was soon going to have them moving the glasses into the next room. Our perplexity about the implausibility of such stimulation doing anything at all led us to feel the need to have the feedback signals analyzed, which led to a private grant to have the system evaluated by Lawrence Livermore Labs (LLNL) in Livermore, California.

Data from an unpublished LLNL (Bland, 2000) analysis of both the I-400 and the I-330 C2, which only became available after the commencement of Kravitz study, showed that the earlier I-400 models of the EEG had no discernable electromagnet field around it, making the LEDs in the glasses the source of the feedback stimulation in the older system (Bland, 2000). However the I-330 C2 generated two different levels of electromagnet field in addition to the light feedback stimulation.

The lowest level of electromagnetic field had strength of 10^{-21} watts/cm². This is the strength of the electromagnetic field while the unit is simply recording data, but not providing feedback–an emission for baseline operation, if you will. The second type of electromagnetic field has strength of 10^{-18} watts/cm².

The generator for these fields was considered by the author of the LLNL (Bland, 2000) study to be the crystal clock in the I-330 C2 that generates the timing signals for the on-board digital signal processor. The digital signal processor provides the capability of much faster analysis of signals than did the desktop computer based analysis in the older I-400 system. The I-400 system had no such on-board microprocessor, and was, therefore, electromagnetically much quieter. Furthermore, Lawrence Livermore Labs said that the glasses, masked as such by the black tape, played no part in the stimulation feedback; in fact, they said that the effects from the system came from the radio frequency carrier wave for the feedback frequencies. All wires attached to the EEG were said by the LLNL staff to be antennas; that is, the EEG leads (active, reference, and ground), the cable from the EEG to the computer, and the cable to the glasses were all, in fact, antennas conducting the electromagnetic field.

Even with the field strength reduced by the radio frequency filters, it still proved somewhat tricky to conduct treatment with very sensitive patients. With the field strength lowered, I began to be bothered by what still seemed to be feedback stimulation that was too intense.

Because I could not remove the radio frequencies which were part and parcel of how the EEG system now operated, in desperation and holding my breath, I disconnected the glasses from the EEG by unplugging the glasses cable. Surprisingly, the system still worked–and worked better. The EEG leads remained the effective source of the radio frequencies once the cable to the glasses was removed. This, then, is the configuration we finally settled on with the I-330 C2, and used in treatment until still newer generations of equipment were produced by J&J with 3,000 to 4,000 times less electromagnetic field strength. In fact, we no longer needed the heavy electromagnetic field filters with the newer equipment. We have found, however, that we still need to continue the process of giving only seconds of feedback in any one session. By the time we discovered that we needed to eliminate the glasses, however, the Kravitz study, with the greater intensity electromagnetic field, was either well under way or had completed the running of participants.

In summary, the EEG preamplifier used in the Kravitz study emitted a hitherto unknown radio frequency stimulus that was strong enough to reduce the efficacy of the feedback system. This caused temporary side effects such as fatigue and interfered with the reduction of symptoms. This stimulation was not present in the previous generations of equipment, and is vastly reduced in intensity in the current models–reduced enough to not be a problem as long as we keep the feedback exposure short with most of the clinical conditions with which we now work. In conclusion, while there may be other factors that encumbered the efficacy of FNS in the study, it seems to me that the electromagnetic field, in general, but particularly from the glasses cable, was the primary reason that the Kravitz study did not succeed. This seems supported by our clinical experiences where we found the need to avoid using the cable and glasses in working with patients.

REFERENCES

Bland, M. F. (2000). *Electromagnetic emission from I-400, C2 high power and C2 low power glasses.* Unpublished report, Livermore, CA: Lawrence Livermore National Laboratory.

Donaldson, C. C. S., Sella, G. E., & Mueller, H. H. (1998). Fibromyalgia. A retrospective study of 252 consecutive referrals. *Canadian Journal of Clinical Medicine, 5,* 116-121,124-127.

Kravitz, H. M., Esty, M. L., Katz, R. S., & Fawcett, J. (2006) *Journal of Neurotherapy, 10* (2), 41-58.

Mueller, H., Donaldson, C. S., Nelson, D., Layman, M. (2001). Treatment of Fibromyalgia incorporating EEG-driven stimulation: A clinical outcomes study. *Journal of Clinical Psychology, 57* (7), 933-952.

Schoenberger, N., Shiflett, S., Esty, M. L., Ochs, L., & Matheis, R. J. (2001). Flexyx neurotherapy system in the treatment of traumatic brain injury: An initial evaluation. *Journal of Head Trauma Rehabilitation, 16* (3), 260-274.

doi:10.1300/J184v10n02_04

Reflections on FMS Treatment, Research, and Neurotherapy: Cautionary Tales

Mary Lee Esty, PhD

SUMMARY. Treatment planning for a patient diagnosed with fibromyalgia (FMS) requires neurotherapists to consider a wide range of potential causes during history taking. Effective treatment planning often involves interventions from multiple specialists coordinating treatments. Creation of a treatment team may involve, in addition to neurotherapy, medical specialties such as infectious disease, physical medicine, neurology, nutrition, and rheumatology, as well as cranial sacral and myofascial treatments, and surface electromyography (sEMG). Understanding the signs of common complications in those diagnosed with FMS is vital to effective treatment. doi:10.1300/J184v10n02_05 *[Article copies available for a fee from The Haworth Document Delivery Service: 1-800-HAWORTH. E-mail address: <docdelivery@haworthpress.com> Website: <http://www.HaworthPress.com> © 2006 by The Haworth Press, Inc. All rights reserved.]*

KEYWORDS. Neurotherapy, fibromyalgia, chronic fatigue syndrome, chronic pain, chronic infection, myofascial pain

Lessons learned from the experiences of subjects in the Rush-Presbyterian-St. Luke's Medical Center and Neurotherapy Center of Washington fibromyalgia study (Kravitz, Esty, Katz & Fawcett, 2006) provide a rich and evolving store of information for neurotherapists treating anyone diagnosed with fibromyalgia (FMS). The coexisting conditions described below are not proven causes of FMS, even though it is often tempting to make that assumption. However, making such a link is a task that will require more research. Nonetheless, an appreciation of common complications often accompanying the FMS diagnostic label is essential to good treatment planning. This note is offered as supplementary information that may be helpful to therapist and patient alike.

Getting clear and reliable research results with people diagnosed with FMS is very difficult. The official criteria for this diagnosis were established for research purposes in 1990 as a result of a consensus conference (Wolfe et al., 1990). Two groups of doctors evaluated patients who had been diagnosed by physicians considered experts on the condition. The resulting consensus opinion, arrived at independently between the two groups, was that all of the patients expertly diagnosed with FMS exhibited 11 of 18 tender points in selected sites on

Mary Lee Esty is affiliated with the Neurotherapy Center of Washington, 5480 Wisconsin Avenue, Suite 221, Chevy Chase, MD 20815 (E-mail: info@neurotherapycenters.com).

[Haworth co-indexing entry note]: "Reflections on FMS Treatment, Research, and Neurotherapy: Cautionary Tales." Esty, Mary Lee. Co-published simultaneously in *Journal of Neurotherapy* (The Haworth Medical Press, an imprint of The Haworth Press, Inc.) Vol. 10, No. 2/3, 2006, pp. 63-68; and: *LENS: The Low Energy Neurofeedback System* (ed: D. Corydon Hammond) The Haworth Medical Press, an imprint of The Haworth Press, Inc., 2006, pp. 63-68. Single or multiple copies of this article are available for a fee from The Haworth Document Delivery Service [1-800-HAWORTH, 9:00 a.m. - 5:00 p.m. (EST). E-mail address: docdelivery@haworthpress.com].

the body. This work, which was originally intended only for use in a single study, became the standard for diagnosing FMS.

Full discussion of the difficulties with these criteria would be lengthy and inconclusive. The important point here is that diagnosis of FMS is complicated. FMS is a condition that appears to have multiple causations, a complex interplay and mix of psychophysiological dysfunctions, soft tissue damage, physical and emotional trauma, infectious agents, toxic exposure, and genetic syndromes. Some of the Rush study participants (Kravitz et al., 2006) had a combination of these problems. The resulting variety of symptoms that can be present in one person makes treatment planning a challenge. The remainder of this paper discusses different etiologic factors that may be involved with the various subtypes of FMS and their implications for treatment.

CENTRAL NERVOUS SYSTEM FACTORS

As a result of following some of the subjects in the Rush study even after the study ended, the Neurotherapy Center of Washington therapists came to a deeper understanding of the frustrations of patients and clinicians alike. Despite current research establishing that people diagnosed with FMS are suffering from a central nervous system (CNS) problem, there is still a perception among some health care providers that it is a psychosomatic problem and that psychotherapy is the treatment of choice. One leading FMS researcher states that FMS is a distinct clinical syndrome deserving of informed medical care and continued research to better understand chronic widespread pain (Russell, 1999). Staud, Price et al. (2001) report that pain ratings in response to a heat stimulus are greater in fibromyalgia subjects as compared to controls, providing evidence for central abnormal pain modulation controls. Staud, Caril et al. (2001) write that "FMS subjects required much lower mechanical pressures than controls to elicit wind-up, indicating abnormal pain mechanisms. These same mechanisms may also play an important role in FMS pain" (p. 79). Wittrup et al. (2001) looked at markers of CNS injury through measures of inflammatory markers in cerebrospinal fluid and serum. They found an immuno-inflammatory process in the CNS that supports "a model of immune-mediated brain injury leading to abnormal sensory processing and widespread allodynia in FMS" (Wittrup et al., 2001; p. 81). They also suggest that their findings support subgrouping FMS patients by etiology.

Of particular interest to neurotherapists is research from brain scans. Using SPECT scanning, Mountz (2002) identified decreased blood flow in the thalamus and caudate nucleus. These are areas that generally modulate pain signals. The research group concluded that "... specific parts of the brain's limbic system, the thalamus and caudate nucleus, have decreased blood flow. These areas seem to modulate pain by inhibiting incoming pain signals. If they are not functioning normally, they will not be able to inhibit pain signals. Fibromyalgia seems to 'turn off' these areas, which allows pain signals to continue uninhibited through the brain" (p. 38).

Based on my clinical experience over the last decade with many FMS patients, it is difficult to agree with the suggestion that fibromyalgia is the cause of a change in brain function. Given what is now known from QEEG, imaging data, and patient histories, trauma of some type has changed the brain's functioning and *this is the biomechanical contribution to the onset* of fibromyalgia symptoms. The thalamic area of the brain is especially vulnerable to physical damage from blunt and whiplash trauma. The sella turcica (Turkish saddle) is the bony cavity in which the pituitary gland is encased. The pituitary stalk passes through a small opening leading to the hypothalamus. This cozy little dwelling is highly protective of the master gland, but the design has a significant drawback to overall functioning following any head trauma involving acceleration or deceleration. When any momentum causes the head to be accelerated or decelerated, the brain, suspended in fluid, bounces in relation to the forces involved, or is twisted in any rotational event such as a car spinning. The result is a stretching of the pituitary stalk and interference with hormone functions in which the pituitary is a key player (Silverman, 2002). The pituitary is responsible for regulating hormones that affect many organ systems. Thyroid, sex and adrenal hormone problems are only a few issues that can follow trauma to this part of the brain.

Donaldson, Donaldson, Mueller, and Sella (2003) identified sub-groups in fibromyalgia based upon quantitative EEG (QEEG) brainwave patterns. This research points to a significant CNS component in FMS. Perhaps, as they suggest, there is an EEG signature in people with fibromyalgia. Schwartz and Begley (2002) provide a lively and well-documented history of research on the mechanisms and applications for treatments based on neuroplasticity and give hopeful news about the ability of the brain to change in response to stimulation.

An increased understanding of the role of brain function on pain and on chronic illnesses is appearing more frequently in pain research literature. Researchers (Tennant, 2003) presenting at the American Pain Society and the American Academy of Pain Medicine reported, ". . . clear evidence that chronic pain produces cardiovascular and immunologic complications. Even more compelling was a study by Sora and Associates from Northwestern University that compared brain mass in chronic pain patients with normal controls. The chronic pain patients' gray matter had significantly less density . . . Although nervous system-type pain, per se, is in early stages of research, practitioners and patients need to be keenly aware that there is growing evidence that uncontrolled pain may produce pathologic, neurologic, immunologic, cardiovascular and endocrine changes" (p. 8).

Neurotherapy

Even if the CNS dysfunction factor of FMS etiology is accepted, does it follow that treatment to correct only the CNS contribution to the syndrome is sufficient for recovery? It is my belief that treatment of CNS dysfunction is an essential component of any treatment plan for recovery from the symptoms of FMS, but in most cases it is not sufficient. Neurotherapy will be most successful in those who were functioning well prior to a physically traumatic onset. It will not produce significant change in those with ongoing infection, significant toxic exposure, or structural damage. Complicated psychological trauma is another complication, as are genetic syndromes.

As neurotherapists accept the challenge to improve the CNS functioning of people diagnosed with FMS, the body must not be forgotten. Soft tissue and structural problems, as well as endocrinological issues caused by biomechanical forces of head trauma, must be addressed directly. Infectious agents are often a constant drain on energy and nutrition, and they may have entered the CNS. All of these problems must be detected and properly treated to maximize clinical benefits. Some case examples illustrate common problems presented by FMS patients.

INFECTION

D is a 51-year-old woman who entered the Rush study at age 46. She was in the placebo group first, and had no positive response, but had some significant, but not complete, relief from the active treatment. There was improvement, but she still had some symptoms even after some post-study FNS treatment. She returned for more treatment in late 2005 with pain all-over, aching, and cognitive fogginess. Surface EMG (sEMG) evaluation revealed 8 imbalances of 13 muscles tested, many of them extreme imbalances. Response to the EEG stimulation treatment led to rapid improvement in cognitive functioning. Three sEMG treatment sessions gave her some tools that diminished pain a bit, but nothing helped with the aching. She was recently diagnosed with Lyme disease and has just begun treatment. Her partial response to treatments is typical of those who have a chronic infection.

Irritable bowel syndrome, ulcerative colitis, and infections such as mycoplasmas, herpes, chlamydia and Lyme disease are common in those with FMS diagnoses. These conditions will make treatment response guarded at best. As an example, Dennis and Bright (2003) wrote a paper on treating fungal sinusitis. They had collected data on 624 patients treated over 14 years with diagnoses of fibromyalgia, chronic fatigue syndrome (CFS), arthritis, and other immune diseases. These patients were treated with medications, surgery where indicated, and environmental cleanup to specific standards of fungal presence. "Neurofeedback was attempted without success before environmental cleanup was accomplished" (p. 89). The conclusion was that wellness and effective neurotherapy can be achieved only *after* appropriate interventions targeting the infectious process are completed.

Nicolson et al. (2000) has done extensive research on the nature of Gulf War Illness, documenting the difficulty of differentiating FMS from CFS and rheumatoid arthritis. They concluded:

Bacterial and viral infections are associated with many chronic illnesses as causative agents, cofactors or more likely as opportunistic infections in immune suppressed individuals. The prevalence of invasive pathogenic *Mycoplasma* species infections (and possibly other bacterial infections, such as *Chlamydia, Borrelia,* etc.) in patients with Chronic Fatigue Syndrome, Fibromyalgia Syndrome, Gulf War Illness, Rheumatoid Arthritis and other chronic illnesses was significantly higher than in healthy controls. When we examined chronic illness patients for multiple *Mycoplasma* species infections, we found that almost all patients had multiple intracellular infections, suggesting that multiple bacterial infections commonly occur in certain chronic illness patients. These patients generally respond to particular antibiotics if administered long-term, but an important part of their recovery involves nutritional supplementation with appropriate vitamins, minerals, immune enhancement and other supplements. Nutraceuticals appear to be necessary for recovery and maintenance of a strong immune system. In addition, patients should be removed from potentially immune-depressing drugs, such as some antidepressants, to allow recovery of their immune systems. Other chronic infections (viral) may also be involved in various chronic fatigue illnesses with or without mycoplasmal and other bacterial infections, and these multiple infections could be important in causing patient morbidity and resulting difficulties in treating these illnesses. (p. 89)

Viral infection can even exist inside muscles. One recent report (Douche-Aourik et al., 2003) concluded that, "Enterovirus RNA has been found previously in specimens of muscle biopsy from patients with idiopathic dilated cardiomyopathy, chronic inflammatory muscle diseases, and fibromyalgia or chronic fatigue syndrome (fibromyalgia/chronic fatigue syndrome). These results suggest that skeletal muscle may host enteroviral persistent infection" (p. 47).

PARASITES AND CHRONIC PAIN

A parasitic gastrointestinal infection can cause extreme soft tissue pain. A clinical example was found in one 23-year-old patient who had a parasitic infection that caused inflammation of the descending colon that lead to inflammation of the tissues around the left hip with swelling and intense pain. Inflammation of the transverse colon leads to inflammation of surrounding soft tissues such as the genitofemoral, lateral femoral cutaneous and femoral nerves, and the fascia connecting the diaphragm to the T12 area of the spine. Inflammation of these structures sets up a cycle of nerve irritation, swelling, compression, reduced range of motion, and increased nerve irritation. The effects are widespread causing pain even with proper breathing and normal movement, resulting in more bracing against pain, leading to more constriction of movement, increased irritation and inflammation. Breaking this cycle requires elimination of the infection followed by myofascial release and re-education of body mechanics. Detection and diagnosis of some of these infections can be a complicated process but is the necessary first step of a treatment plan.

GENETIC SYNDROMES

Ehlers-Danlos Syndrome (EDS), a genetic condition, is sometimes found in patients diagnosed with fibromyalgia. EDS is a rare hereditary connective tissue disorder characterized by unusually flexible joints, very elastic skin and fragile soft tissue. The skin can be stretched several inches and yet retain its original shape on release. People with this syndrome bruise easily, have a lot of sprains and dislocation of joints, bleed easily, and may have hernias. There is no fully effective treatment, but some physical therapy can strengthen tendons around the joints. A mistaken diagnosis of FMS is understandable for people with EDS because the nature of the tissues creates a vulnerability to injuries from many of life's ordinary activities.

Another genetic condition that can complicate treatment of FMS is von Willebrand's Disease (vWD). It involves a deficiency of a protein that affects platelet function, resulting in slowed cessation of bleeding. Platelets that should form the first step in repairing a cut are not active, so bleeding does not stop quickly. People with vWD bruise easily, and bleed excessively after a cut or from dental work. Recovery from any invasive procedure is prolonged, and even a colonoscopy can be physically traumatic. Fatigue from iron deficiency becomes a problem.

STRUCTURAL INJURIES

Acceleration and deceleration forces wreak exquisite damage on the brain's internal structures leading to cognitive dysfunctions of memory and attention as well as to the inability of the brain to properly handle noxious stimuli, including vestibular problems. Structural damage resulting from physical trauma is often involved in the onset of FMS. Severe coccyx injury from a fall onto the tailbone often occurs during stairway accidents, or from sports activities. This can be a cause of chronic headache. Whiplash can cause a reversal of normal curvature of the spine (cervical lordosis). This causes extreme pain and requires skilled physical therapy.

Motor vehicle accidents are the most common cause of traumatic brain injury, and whiplash is a commonly reported as a precipitating cause of FMS. The effects of whiplash extend far beyond the muscle damage that causes headache and the neck/back spasms that can lead to chronic pain. Damage to the central nervous system results from physical forces on the brain inside the skull. "Wherever there is momentum, there is a potential for tissue injury. Whenever a whiplash injury occurs, there is a

risk for chronic painful complications such as fibromyalgia" (Pellegrino, 2002; p. 14).

Brown (2001) documented G forces to the brain resulting from low-speed rear-end collisions. In the first 100 milliseconds after collision, the car moves from under the body and the torso rises. The forces involved are compression, torsion, and shear. It is the compression and shear that cause big problems. In 200 milliseconds the head starts back and rises. Between 200 to 300 milliseconds later, the body starts forward–even faster than it went backward–but the head always lags behind, and then whips forward. One hundred milliseconds after a 20 mph impact, the acceleration inside the skull reaches 18Gs. "The most important factor regarding motor vehicle collisions and injuries is how much (or how little) of the collision force is absorbed by the occupants" (Pellegrino, 2002; p. 3).

VESTIBULAR DAMAGE

Serious vestibular problems can result from head trauma and be coexistent with the FMS diagnosis. These must be taken very seriously because the condition affects all treatment of these patients, neurotherapy as well as sEMG. A clinical example illustrates the need for careful treatment planning to avoid undue use of resources.

One patient responded well to FNS with improvement in the cognitive area. Treatment of the muscle imbalances was temporarily helpful, but would not hold. She had inner ear damage that interpreted an off-center posture as being balanced. This kept the muscles in chronically stressful positions that reinforced muscle imbalances and pain. This condition must be repaired. Many of these people require treatment for benign paroxysmal positional vertigo.

Another dysfunction that can result from biomechanical trauma is a perilymphatic fistula, an opening in the inner ear that causes severe dizziness. It can sometimes be repaired surgically. Another patient responded with improvement in cognitive functioning, but the pain persisted. She had a serious fall on the tailbone that was responsible for continuing pain. Appropriate myofascial treatment has been helpful in reducing pain. Such falls are often a factor in chronic headache.

CONCLUSION

In summary, taking the history of people diagnosed with FMS should delve into great detail about head trauma and past illnesses that were not usually considered significant at the time. This meticulous investigation is important even though thorough attention to the details of their history and symptoms can seem somewhat tangential to their main concerns. Involvement of proper specialists is then required. Neurotherapy alone will often not help these people.

REFERENCES

Brown, C. R. (2001, September). *Injury, biomechanical trauma and forensic practice.* Paper presented at the American Academy of Pain Management Conference, Alexandria, VA.

Dennis, D., & Bright, G. (2003). Treating fungal sinusitis. [Abstract]. *Journal of Neurotherapy, 8* (4), 88-89.

Donaldson M., Donaldson, C. C. S., Mueller, H. H., & Sella, G. (2003). QEEG patterns, psychological status, and pain reports of fibromyalgia sufferers. *American Journal of Pain Management, 13* (2), 60-73.

Douche-Aourik F., Perlier W., Feasson, L., Bourlet T., Harrath, R., Omar, S. et al. (2003). *Journal of Medical Virology, 71* (4), 540-547.

Kravitz, H. M., Esty, M. L., Katz, R. S., & Fawcett, J. (2006). Treatment of fibromyalgia syndrome using low-intensity neurofeedback with the Flexyx neurotherapy system: A randomized controlled clinical trial. *Journal of Neurotherapy, 10* (2/3), 41-58.

Mountz, J. M. (2002). Fibromyalgia in women: Abnormalities of regional cerebral blood flow in the thalamus and caudate nucleus are associated with low pain threshold levels. In M. Pelligrino (Ed.), *Whiplash to fibromyalgia* (p. 74). North Canton, OH: ORC Publications.

Nicolson, G. L., Nasralla, M. Y., Franco, A. R., DeMeirleir, K., Nicolson, N. L. Ngwenya, R., et al. (2000). Role of mycoplasmal infections in fatigue illnesses: Chronic fatigue and fibromyalgia syndromes, Gulf war illness and rheumatoid arthritis. *Journal of Chronic Fatigue Syndrome, 6* (3/4), 23-29.

Pellegrino, M. J. (2002). *From whiplash to fibromyalgia.* North Canton, OH: ORC Publications.

Russell, I. J. (1999). Is fibromyalgia a distinct clinical entity? The clinical investigator's evidence. *Baillieres Best Practice in Research Clinical Rheumatology, 13* (3), 445-454.

Schwartz, J., & Begley, S. (2002). *The mind and the brain.* New York: Regan Books, Harper Collins.

Silverman, S. (2002, April). Orofacial and pharyngeal disorders associated with traumatic brain injury. Presentation at the New York Academy of Traumatic Brain Injury Conference, NYU School of Medicine, New York City.

Staud, R., Caril, K., Vierck, C. J., Price, D. D., Robinson, M., Canon, R., et al. (2001). Mechanical muscle stimuli result in enhanced temporal summation of second pain [wind-up] in fibromyalgia subjects. [Abstract] *Journal of Musculoskeletal Pain, 9,* 79.

Staud, R., Price, D. D., Vierck, C. J., Dloughy, B., Cannon, R., & Robinson, M. (2001). Diffuse noxious inhibitory controls [DMIC] do not inhibit wind-up of fibromyalgia patients. [Abstract] *Journal of Musculoskeletal Pain, 9,* 78.

Tennant, F. (2003). Time to be more aggressive. Editorial. *Practical Pain Management, 3,* 8.

Wittrup, I., Christiansen, M., Jensen, B., Bliddal, H., Danneskiold-Samsoe, B., Wiik, A. (2001). Markers of central nervous system injury in two cohorts of patients with fibromyalgia. [Abstract] *Journal of Musculoskeletal Pain, 9,* 81.

Wolfe, F., Smythe, H. A., Yunus, M. B., Bennett, R. M., Bombardier, C., & Goldenberg, D. L. (1990). The American College of Rheumatology 1990 criteria for the classification of fibromyalgia. (Report of the Multicenter Criteria Committee.) *Arthritis and Rheumatism, 33,* 160-172.

doi:10.1300/J184v10n02_05

The LENS (Low Energy Neurofeedback System): A Clinical Outcomes Study on One Hundred Patients at Stone Mountain Center, New York

Stephen Larsen, PhD
Kristen Harrington, MA
Susan Hicks, BA

SUMMARY. *Introduction.* The Low Energy Neurofeedback System (LENS) developed by Dr. Len Ochs (2006a) uses feedback in the form of a radio frequency carrier wave, administered at a positive *offset* frequency from the person's own dominant EEG frequency. Although it is an unusual biofeedback procedure, the feedback being invisible and the subject passive, clinical evidence supports the efficacy of the LENS across a spectrum of conditions. Published research studies (Schoenberger, Shifflet, Esty, Ochs, & Matheis, 2001; Donaldson, Sella, & Mueller, 1998; Mueller, Donaldson, Nelson, & Layman, 2001) have shown the effectiveness of the LENS method with traumatic brain injury (TBI) and with fibromyalgia. No study to date has evaluated LENS treatment across the spectrum of disorders and with a significantly large sample. This study was devised to address these issues. The study hypotheses were that the LENS treatment would be effective in reducing both systematic symptom ratings and measurements of EEG amplitudes, and that the therapeutic effect would produce the most rapid improvements in early sessions of treatment.

Method. "Blinded" research associates selected the first 100 patients from approximately 300 case files that met the following inclusion criteria: the person had received at least 10 treatment sessions, completed an initial CNS questionnaire, and that session-by-session subjective symptom ratings (SSRF) had been obtained. Patients ranged from 6 to 80 years old, almost evenly divided between male and female, with a wide range of symptoms and comorbid DSM-IV diagnoses.

Results. Data were statistically analyzed for significance and corelational variables. Average symptom ratings across 15 major problem areas (e.g., anxiety, mood disturbance, attentional problems, fatigue, pain, sleep problems, etc.) showed significant improvements ($p < .0001$) from beginning to end of treatment. After an average of only 20 treatments the mean average of patient symptom ratings (0-10) declined from 7.92 to 3.96, a 50% improvement. Equally significant was the drop in EEG amplitude at the highest amplitude electrode site (HAS; $p < .0001$) as well as a lesser but still significant decrease at Cz ($p < .002$). A final analysis of the average symptom score with the HAS score showed them to be highly correlated. All hypotheses were confirmed.

Stephen Larsen is Psychology Professor Emeritus at SUNY, and Director of the Stone Mountain Center.

Kristen Harrington is a Licensed Marriage and Family Therapist and is affiliated with the Stone Mountain Center.

Susan Hicks is a Mathematical Statistician.

Address correspondence to: Stephen Larsen, Stone Mountain Center, 475 River Road Extension, New Paltz, NY 12561 (E-mail: office@stonemountaincenter.com).

The authors acknowledge Alexandra Linardakis, BA, Jodie Schultz, MA, and Tara Johannessen, BA, research assistants on this project.

[Haworth co-indexing entry note]: "The LENS (Low Energy Neurofeedback System): A Clinical Outcomes Study on One Hundred Patients at Stone Mountain Center, New York." Larsen, Stephen, Kristen Harrington, and Susan Hicks. Co-published simultaneously in *Journal of Neurotherapy* (The Haworth Medical Press, an imprint of The Haworth Press, Inc.) Vol. 10, No. 2/3, 2006, pp. 69-78; and: *LENS: The Low Energy Neurofeedback System* (ed: D. Corydon Hammond) The Haworth Medical Press, an imprint of The Haworth Press, Inc., 2006, pp. 69-78. Single or multiple copies of this article are available for a fee from The Haworth Document Delivery Service [1-800-HAWORTH, 9:00 a.m. - 5:00 p.m. (EST). E-mail address: docdelivery@haworthpress.com].

Available online at http://jn.haworthpress.com
doi:10.1300/J184v10n02_06

Conclusions. LENS treatment appears to be very efficient and effective in rapidly reducing a wide range of symptoms. It particularly produces rapid improvements in the first five to six sessions. Recommendations for future research are provided. doi:10.1300/J184v10n02_06 *[Article copies available for a fee from The Haworth Document Delivery Service: 1-800-HAWORTH. E-mail address: <docdelivery@haworthpress.com> Website: <http://www.HaworthPress.com> © 2006 by The Haworth Press, Inc. All rights reserved.]*

KEYWORDS. Neurofeedback, EEG biofeedback, LENS, Low Energy Neurofeedback System

INTRODUCTION

The LENS

The Low Energy Neurofeedback System (LENS), devised by Dr. Len Ochs and tested by him and clinicians he has trained, has evolved continuously for 16 years (Ochs, 2006a). This neurofeedback system provides the patient with instantaneous electromagnetic field feedback that is "offset" by 5, 10, 15, or 20 Hz faster than the patient's dominant brainwave frequency to avoid any possibility of seizures being triggered by the procedure. While treatment relied on flashing lights in the past, a technical laboratory examination of the equipment showed the effective mechanism of treatment to be carried on radio frequency waves of extremely low intensity (Ochs, 2006b) and at 15-100m Hz frequency range.

Len Ochs (1994) had claimed to often obtain very significant improvements with many patients in less than ten sessions. This sometimes raised eyebrows and skepticism among colleagues in the field of neurofeedback. Nonetheless anecdotal experiences by trained LENS practitioners, including the authors, had confirmed the tenor of his claims. In addition, a growing body of published literature (Donaldson, Sella, & Mueller, 1998; Larsen, 2006; Mueller, Donaldson, Nelson, & Layman, 2001; Schoenberger, Shiflett, Esty, Ochs, & Matheis, 2001) had shown that the LENS was effective in ameliorating a variety of conditions associated with CNS dysfunction. What seemed unanswered was whether the LENS procedure produced more effective results early in treatment compared with later? Did all problems respond equally well, or some problems respond better and some worse than others? Therefore, the authors decided to gather data on the effects of LENS treatment in clinical office cases. This paper reports our findings.

The authors began several years ago to systematically collect assessment and outcome data on clinical cases that we treated. In each case, during the intake interview, patients completed the CNS Questionnaire (see Appendix) developed by Ochs (1996, 2006a). After completing the questionnaire patient were asked: "Of these reported symptoms/problem areas, which most impair your quality of life?" The problems of greatest concern were then listed first on our Subjective Symptom Reporting Scale (SSRS), followed by others, until five or more symptoms were elicited and entered. Each was rated by the patient on a 0 to 10 scale. They were told, "Ten (10) means the worst possible interference with your freedom, creativity, and ability to enjoy life; Zero (0) means the problem has disappeared or become unnoticeable." The therapist and the patient agreed to work collaboratively to track these numbers and their ratings were obtained at the beginning of every session. If the patient was a child, a parent or guardian was asked to help with the evaluation ratings. If a spouse or partner attended the treatment session, they were asked to help confirm the veracity of the answer–a "second opinion." Sometimes a symptom might have fluctuated over the week. For example, insomnia may have varied from 2 (a pretty good night) to a 6 (a much worse night's sleep) as reported on the SSRS rating form. In such cases, an average number for the period since the last session (e.g., the number 4, in our example) would to be entered for that period.

This study consists of a retrospective analysis of the five most serious symptoms reported by patients from the beginning to completion of treatment. Figure 1 displays examples of average symptom ratings that were obtained over

FIGURE 1. Progress of an "Easy" Care and a Difficult Case

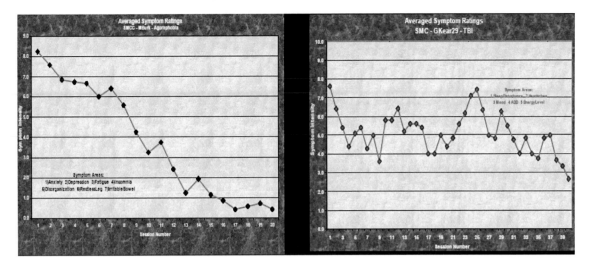

the course of treatment with a relatively "easy" case that responded rapidly, and with a more difficult case that responded to treatment more gradually.

METHOD

Sample

As indicated, our subjects were not specially selected experimental subjects. They were patients who came for treatment between 2001 and 2005 at our offices in New Paltz, New York City, Long Island, and Kingston, New York. Approximately half of the patients were physician-referred. The sample ranged in age from age 6 to age 80 (see the distribution in Figure 2), with the majority of the sample between age 11 and 60 and fairly evenly divided between male and female. The majority of patients received LENS treatment on a weekly basis, but a few were treated twice weekly at the beginning, and then toward the end of treatment most patients were weaned off treatment with semi-weekly or monthly sessions.

Sampling Procedure

From a sample of about three hundred patient files, 100 cases were randomly selected for retrospective examination by blinded research associates who knew nothing about the patients

personally. The research associates signed a form agreeing to protect patient privacy and the actual names were masked and a code name assigned to each file. No attempt was made to select "good responders" or "poor responders" to treatment. Simply the first 100 cases that met the following criteria were chosen for study. The file qualified for inclusion in the study if it had:

1. An initial LENS topographic brain map. Once selected, from these maps the microvolt amplitudes were obtained for the highest amplitude site (HAS) and for the Cz electrode site.
2. The patient had received 10 or more clinical treatment sessions with the LENS.
3. An intake CNS Questionnaire and initial symptom ratings had been completed for at least five symptoms, and symptom rating data had been gathered for at least 10 sessions.
4. Measurements of the overall EEG amplitudes at Cz and the HAS had been completed at the final treatment session.

Hypotheses

The following hypotheses were examined to explore how observations by Len Ochs and others clinicians would stand up to systematic assessment across a variety of symptom areas.

FIGURE 2. Distribution of Clients by Age

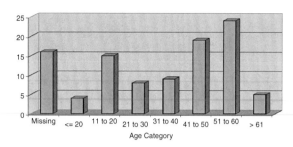

Age Category

- Lens treatment (independent variable) will improve quality of life (dependent variable) across a variety of CNS-related symptom areas as reflected in the Subjective Symptom Rating Scale (Larsen, 2001).
- There will be a steady improvement in symptoms throughout treatment, but improvement will be most noticeable in the early sessions.
- There will be a decrease in overall EEG amplitudes over treatment at the highest amplitude site (HAS) and at the vertex (Cz) as measured on a LENS topographic map.
- There will be a correlation between subjective ratings of symptom improvement and an objective physiological measure of EEG amplitude as measured in microvolt levels.

In relation to the third hypothesis, it should be noted that Ochs (2006a) has suggested that cortical EEG amplitudes are highest where the cortex is functioning most poorly in inhibiting subcortical activity. The topographic map used in LENS practice, with its accompanying histogram (see Ochs, 2006a for an example) quantifies measures taken at 19 or more electrode sites. Based on our clinical experience, we predicted the HAS would decrease in amplitude as treatment rendered the cortex more functional.

Measures and Symptomatic Complaints

As indicated, ratings were examined on the Subjective Symptom Rating Scale (SSRS) and EEG amplitude measures were obtained. On the SSRS we used the patient's own descriptive terms such as "fatigue," "moodiness," "mental cloudiness," etc. Many patients were tracked on as many as eight to ten symptoms, but for the purposes of this study we selected only the five most significant symptoms.

After examination of the data 15 categories were developed to which all of the symptoms reported in the study could be assigned: Addiction (alcohol, drugs, food, sex), Anxiety Problem (generalized anxiety disorder, panic attacks, phobias, hypervigilance), Attention Problem (ADD/ADHD, problems concentrating), Cognitive Problem (cloudiness, cognitive deficit, memory problems, confusion), Dissociation (dissociated, detached, withdrawn), Disorganization (disorganized, procrastination), Problem in Executive Function (impaired planning, sequencing, impulsiveness), Pain, Fatigue (lack of energy, chronic fatigue, fibromyalgia), Flexibility Problem (rigidity or obsessive-compulsive disorder), Mood Disturbance (dysthymia, depression, bipolar disorder, irritability, explosiveness), Sleep Disturbance (insomnia, early morning awakening, restless legs), and a Miscellaneous category for less frequently encountered symptoms (tics, seizures, psychotic symptoms). The distribution of symptoms by category in our sample may be seen in Figure 3. It can be observed that the mostly highly represented problem areas were mood disturbance, followed by problems with cognition, pain, disorganization, sleep, anxiety, attention, and fatigue. Although most patients qualified for multiple diagnoses, the complexity of problems in the patient sample may be seen in Figure 4.

Equipment

All treatment was rendered on J&J I-330 C2 or mini-C2 EEG processors with a sampling rate of 1,028 samples per second, using the electromagnetic emissions of their crystal clock, offset at a faster frequency from the dominant brainwave frequency. All treatment used Ochs Labs proprietary versions of J&J's USE 2 or USE 3 software to administer the stimulations. Maps and offset assessments were processed on Ochs Labs proprietary Report Generator.

All treatment followed an initial brain map at 19 or 21 sites, mapping each site individually and processing the map and histogram for delta, theta, alpha and beta frequency bands, along with a measure of total amplitude and dominant frequency maps and histograms. Where it was possible to do an Offset assessment (meaning the patient was *not too* neurologically sensitive) this was done. If an Offset assessment could not be obtained because the patient seemed too hyper-reactive, the default of a +20Hz offset was used. The hardier patients were exposed to somewhere from 1 to 21 seconds of stimulation (10^{-18} watts/sq. cm^2) per session, while patients who were judged to be too sensitive/reactive early in treatment were simply exposed (at least initially) to the background energy level of the system without stimulation, which has been found in laboratory analyses to be only 10^{-21} watts/sq. cm^2 in intensity. The number of treatment sites and seconds of exposure were based on the sensitivity/reactivity of the patient as discussed in Ochs (2006a).

Confounding Factors

About half of our patients come to us on medication prescribed by their physician. Most were informed that they should tell their doctor that they were receiving neurofeedback and releases were signed so that clinicians from our facility could talk to their physicians, neurologists, or psychiatrists. They were advised that during our treatment they might find themselves needing less medication to achieve the same effect, and should they wish to reduce medications, they should do so under the care of their prescribing physician.

Although neurofeedback was, in our estimate, the main therapeutic modality, a proportion of the patients were also treated with photonic stimulation (an infrared stimulation device) for peripheral pain and fatigue syndromes. Several were given instructions in HeartMath (heart rate variability biofeedback). Some took supplements such as B vitamins, glyconutritionals, SAM-e and Rhodiola Rosea. During treatment, patients did in fact often *decrease their prescription medications.* (This measure, in fact, could be a pivotal one to examine in future studies.) We did not control for any of these variables, nor did it seem possible to do so. The only thing that all 100 patients had in common was that they received the LENS treatment for over 10 sessions, and most patients had

20 sessions of LENS treatment (see Figure 5). The mean number of treatment sessions was 19.43 (SD = 5.51). As clinicians, our initial and primary intent in working with these patients was in helping them improve their quality of life and functioning, not conducting a controlled study.

FIGURE 3. Frequency of Complaint by Category

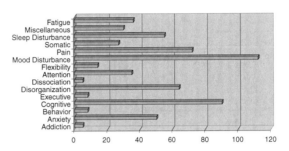

FIGURE 4

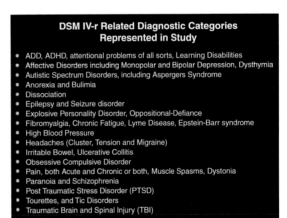

FIGURE 5. Distribution of Number of Treatments

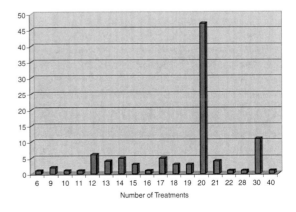

Data Analysis

After gathering and entering data into spreadsheets, the data was compiled and sent to an independent statistician for analysis. Two sample paired t-tests were run on EEG amplitude changes at the HAS and at Cz pre- and post-treatment, and on the average symptom ratings pre- and post-treatment. Logarithmic regressions were then computed on each symptom category to test if the patients were reporting a reduction in symptoms and if that decline was rapid in early treatment sessions.

RESULTS

The results confirmed all hypotheses and the outcomes were found to be highly statistically significant. Every symptom category not only decreased over the course of treatment, demonstrating that LENS treatment was clinically effective in ameliorating widely diverse CNS-related problems, but the second hypothesis was confirmed as well. The decline in the average ratings of symptom categories was found to be greater in early sessions of treatment, with further improvements occurring at a more gradual pace over time, as the experience of Ochs (1994) had suggested. This finding may be seen in Figure 6. It was noted, however, that there was still a definite ongoing continuum of improvement up to 20 sessions and beyond.

In relation to this finding, clinical observations have encouraged us to urge that patients not discontinue LENS treatment after the initial rapid improvements, sometimes called "the honeymoon phase" of treatment because the nervous system continues to gradually reorga-

nize itself. Further treatments beyond the first 10 to 20 sessions may be necessary to consolidate and promote maintenance of the changes achieved early in treatment. Determination of the maintenance of changes over time will require a study with a post-treatment follow-up period.

When each of the 15 symptom categories was plotted by treatment time, it was found that on average the rate of improvement followed a logarithmic curve, with most of the improvements occurring early in treatment, with smaller but steady gains being made thereafter. Although each category appeared slightly different, they all showed the same pattern of rapid improvement with the exception of addiction problems, which was the only symptom category that did not appear responsive to LENS treatment in this study. Figure 7 shows linear regression lines for four sample symptom areas, illustrating what was seen across symptom categories. The r-squared values in rank order of improvement for symptom categories were: Disorganization, .985; Cognitive Problems, .983; Attention, .956; Fatigue, .955; Mood Disturbances, .954; Pain, .941; Anxiety, .928; Executive Function, .903; Miscellaneous Problems, .894; Sleep Disturbances, .891; Somatic Complaints, .874; Flexibility, .864; Behavioral Problems, .857; Dissociation, .715; and Addictions, .0003.

It is evident as seen in Figure 8 that as the length of treatment progresses, particularly beyond 20 sessions (at which point most subjects had completed treatment), the number of observed occurrences of symptoms decreases. Thus beyond 20 sessions and with symptoms that were less frequently represented in the sample, the findings become less reliable as seen in Figure 9. This did not, however, affect the confirmation of the hypotheses of the study which were primarily based on the effect of the first 20 sessions of treatment.

As indicated, the first hypothesis was confirmed by our findings. Figure 10 displays the change during LENS treatment of the mean symptom ratings which, interestingly at post-treatment (3.92) were exactly half of the pre-treatment symptom levels (7.92), a finding that was highly significant (p < .0001).

The third and fourth hypotheses are also confirmed. The overall EEG amplitudes were

FIGURE 6. Plot of Average Score by Treatment All Categories

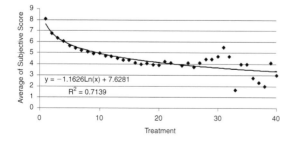

FIGURE 7. Regression Lines for Sample Symptom Categories

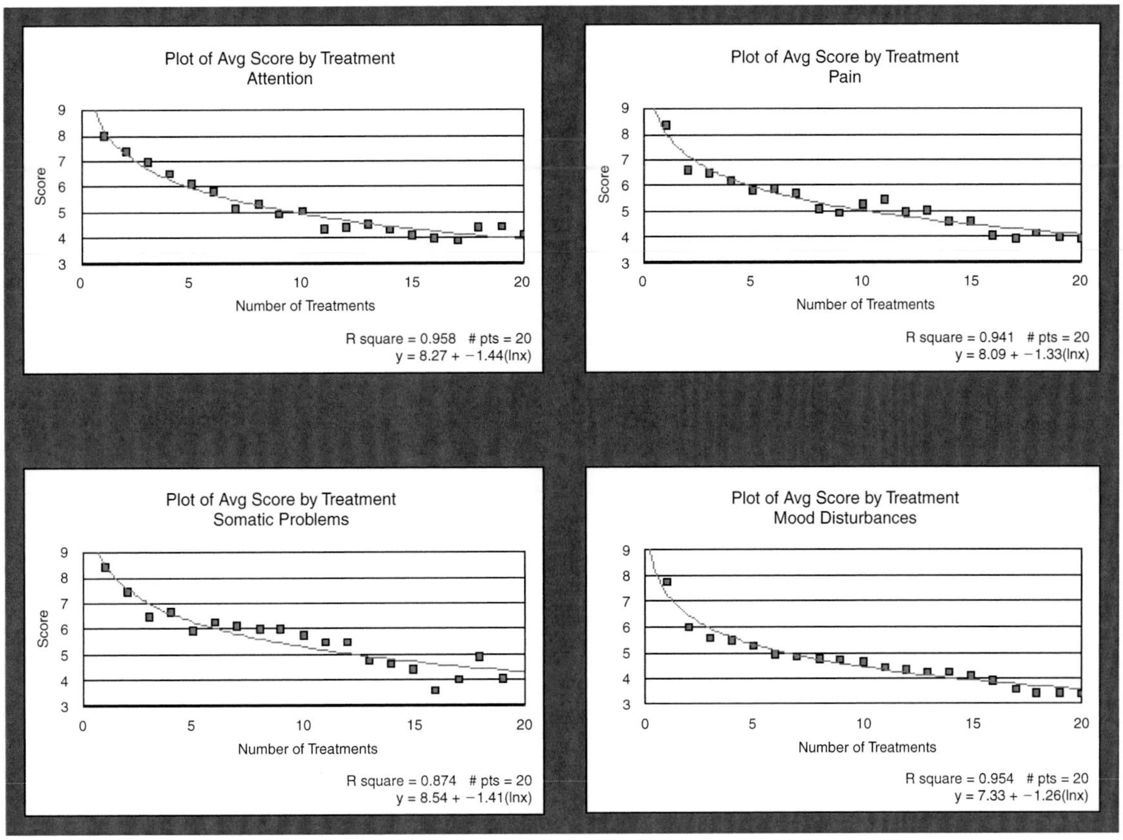

Plot of Avg Score by Treatment
Attention

R square = 0.958   # pts = 20
y = 8.27 + −1.44(lnx)

Plot of Avg Score by Treatment
Pain

R square = 0.941   # pts = 20
y = 8.09 + −1.33(lnx)

Plot of Avg Score by Treatment
Somatic Problems

R square = 0.874   # pts = 20
y = 8.54 + −1.41(lnx)

Plot of Avg Score by Treatment
Mood Disturbances

R square = 0.954   # pts = 20
y = 7.33 + −1.26(lnx)

FIGURE 8. Number of Observations per Treatment Period

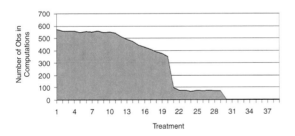

FIGURE 9. 95% Confidence Interval for Change in Scores by Category

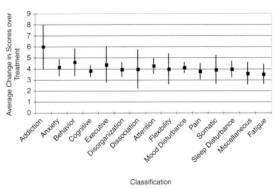

found to significantly (p < .0001) decline over the course of treatments at the highest amplitude site (HAS), as seen in Figure 11. In addition, confirming the fourth hypothesis, this EEG improvement was also highly correlated (r-square = 0.869) with improvements in symptom ratings (as seen in Figure 12). This finding adds validity to the accuracy of the improvements noted in patient self-ratings of their symptoms. Thus, each of the two separate measures, subjective well-being (symptom ratings) and EEG amplitudes, both respond to the independent variable (the LENS treatment).

A significant reduction (p < .0022) in the overall EEG amplitude at Cz was also found, decreasing from 10.67µv to 9.62µv. Since the LENS treatment involved feedback stimula-

FIGURE 10. Average Score Pre- and Post-Treatment

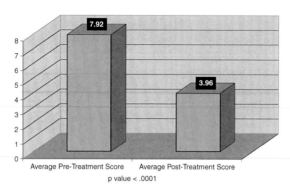

p value < .0001

FIGURE 11. Reduction in Highest Amplitude Size (HAS)

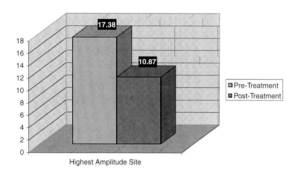

FIGURE 12. Plot of Relative Change in Qualitative Score vs. HAS

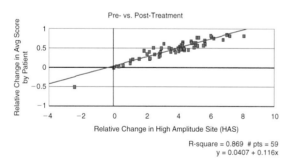

R-square = 0.869 # pts = 59
y = 0.0407 + 0.116x

tion being received at one or more different electrode sites in each session, we had no reason to suspect that activity at CZ would be "treated" more than any other site since, on average, work at Cz occurred only once in about every four to five sessions. However, Cz has often been considered an important site in traditional neurofeedback (Tansey, 1990; Lubar, 1995).

The changes in EEG amplitude at the HAS

provides confirmation of LENS theory (as well as effectiveness). Ochs (2006a) does not believe that LENS treatment will be effective by simply concentrating the treatment in the area of the brain with the highest EEG amplitudes. Interestingly, research (Fernandez et al., 2003) with traditional neurofeedback applied to learning disability children found that the greatest reductions in EEG amplitude often did not occur at the site where neurofeedback treatment was focused. Ochs (2006a) has theorized that by having treatment proceed from locations where there are lower amplitudes toward electrode sites where there are higher amplitudes (which reflect less efficient cortical inhibitory processes) the functioning of the entire cortex will be positively influenced and the amplitudes at the highest amplitude sites will decrease. Such changes had been previously observed in clinical work by Larsen (2001). Though in our current study the HAS would not have received any more treatment emphasis than was received at Cz (as described above) there was found to be an average decrease in amplitudes of 6.51μv at the HAS (see Figure 11). The mean amplitude at the HAS decreased from 17.38μv to 10.84μv, representing a 37% decline.

DISCUSSION

By basing our study on subjective symptoms as described in the patient's own words, we have tried to make this study relevant to people's *quality of life* in a very immediate and practical way. It is true that this type of classification of problems may have made this study superficially seem less technical or professional than a study simply based on strict DSM-IV criteria. However, symptoms are what people suffer with and are the fundamental components that make up diagnostic categories. Whereas many studies through the years have shown limited reliability in assigning diagnostic categories (e.g., Klein, 1982), we believe that symptoms are not only "where people live," but also are more reliably identified in comparison with over-arching diagnoses.

The rationale for tracking five or more symptoms rather than a single one stemmed from the fact that rarely do symptoms exist in isolation. It has also been our clinical observation that improvement is often *a non-linear process*. Thus an individual's presenting complaints may have been anxiety attacks and migraine headaches, but he or she may also complain of problems with fatigue, insomnia, and photophobia. In our clinical work we have noticed in cases like this that the target symptoms of anxiety and migraines may remain approximately the same for a while, while sleep improves and the patient becomes less light-sensitive. These are good signs that seem to indicate that some deeper neurological re-balancing is underway and bodes well for the treatment. Suddenly one day, the patient reports that her schedule is filling up, social anxiety is dwindling, and the migraines are shorter in duration. This is, in fact, not an atypical course of treatment.

Although it would have been ideal in our study to use psychological tests with established validity and reliability because most of our patients had a large number of symptomatic complaints, we made the decision in our office to use symptom ratings at the beginning of each session for accountability. One of the important reasons for this decision was our desire to track session-by-session changes in patient symptoms, in which case it would be impractical to require patients to complete a lengthy psychological test (or multiple tests) once or twice weekly. Therefore, we believed that subjective ratings, particularly when combined with objective physiological (EEG) data, would allow frequent and systematic verification of symptomatic changes. Our results support these decisions.

This study represents an uncontrolled case series. Nonetheless, we believe that the topographic brain map documentation of EEG amplitude changes, and the correlation between these changes and symptom ratings, demonstrate the great likelihood that the changes in our patients did not simply stem from a desire to please a therapist or placebo effects. Therapy was also conducted by four separate therapists.

We should note, in contrast to our present findings, that sometimes in treatment we have found that there may be a rise in EEG amplitudes associated with symptomatic improvements, particularly when the patient has a low voltage EEG at the beginning of treatment. Such a pattern often seems to be associated with

fatigue, depression, lack of motivation, and alcoholism. As the person improves subjectively in such cases, amplitudes go up. Our theory is that in many of these cases, a kind of cortical over-suppression might have been at work, and the therapy restores energy to areas of the brain.

In the kind of clinical cases seen in our study sample, we will also sometimes see the HAS decrease in magnitude, while the lowest amplitude sites come up in microvolts. The net effect is to produce a more balanced looking brain map (site sort), without the bright colors associated with high amplitude activity. Future studies can explore some of these variables.

The rapid improvements found in this study following early LENS treatment sessions has mirrored our clinical experience. We commonly see a rapid decrease in symptoms which then continue to diminish more gradually as treatment progresses through about 20 sessions. It has been our clinical experience that sometimes shortly after patients have received 20 treatment sessions, and leading up to and after 30 sessions, there can sometimes be a surge of symptoms temporarily worsening, followed after about session 33 with the lowest symptom ratings attained. From a clinical perspective, these symptom fluctuations have particularly seemed to be associated with more "chronic" patients whose symptoms are more longstanding and where we believe there is a strong genetic component to the main problem areas (e.g., an affective disorder, or familial ADD). This clinical experience has suggested the hypothesis that continued treatment may possibly be gradually addressing increasing "layers" of CNS dysfunction that did not immediately present themselves or respond readily to initial treatments. These clinical observations support the idea that improvements can continue to occur after a larger number of sessions than was usually administered in this study, perhaps as more "endogenous" factors associated with even deeper levels of CNS functioning are gradually calmed and normalized.

In summary, this study provides further objective evidence for the positive therapeutic outcomes reported by Dr. Len Ochs in previous studies. The results represented therapy conducted by four separate clinicians, following training procedures articulated by Drs. Ochs and Larsen in the training conducted for professionals, providing evidence that the outcomes are not associated with simply a charismatic therapist. It is concluded that LENS provides a very encouraging therapeutic option to traditional neurofeedback for the treatment of a wide range of clinical, brain-related conditions, particularly because LENS requires minimal cooperation and allows the patient to remain passive. It is recommended that future studies employ randomized assignment to LENS treatment in comparison with wait-list control groups, with medication treatment, and that placebo-controlled double-blind studies be done.

REFERENCES

Donaldson, S., Sella, G., & Mueller, H. (1998). Fibromyalgia: A retrospective study of 252 consecutive referrals. *Canadian Journal of Clinical Medicine*, *56*, 116-127.

Fernandez, T., Herrera, W., Harmony, T., Diaz-Comas, L., Santiago, E., Sanchez, L., et al. (2003). EEG and behavioral changes following neurofeedback treatment in learning disabled children. *Clinical Electroencephalography*, *34* (3), 145-150.

Klein, D. N. (1982). Relation between current diagnostic criteria for schizophrenia and the dimensions of premorbid adjustment, paranoid symptomatology, and chronicity. *Journal of Abnormal Psychology*, *91*, 319-325.

Larsen, S., (2001, February). The use of Flexyx treatment modality with patients with multiple brain and spinal cord injuries. Paper presented at Future Health Winter Brain Conference, Miami, FL.

Larsen, S. (2006) *The healing power of neurofeedback*. Rochester, VT: The Healing Arts Press.

Lubar, J. F. (1995). Neurofeedback for the management of attention-deficit/hyperactivity disorders. Chapter in M. S. Schwartz (Ed.), *Biofeedback: A practitioner's guide* (pp. 493-522). New York: Guilford.

Mueller, H. H., Donaldson, C. C. S., Nelson, D. V., & Layman, M. (2001). Treatment of fibromyalgia incorporating EEG-driven stimulation: A clinical outcomes study. *Journal of Clinical Psychology*, *57* (7), 933-952.

Ochs, L. (1994). New light on lights, sounds, and the brain. *Megabrain Report: The Journal of Mind Technology*, *2* (4), 48-52.

Ochs, L. (1996). Thoughts about EEG-Driven stimulation after three years of its uses: Ramifications for concepts of pathology, recovery, and brain function. Unpublished manuscript.

Ochs, L. (2006a). The Low Energy Neurofeedback System (LENS): Theory, Background, and Introduction. *Journal of Neurotherapy*, *10* (2/3), 5-39.

Ochs, L. (2006b). Comment on the Treatment of Fibromyalgia Syndrome Using Low-Intensity Neurofeedback with the Flexyx Neurotherapy System: A Randomized Controlled Clinical Trial; or, How to Go Crazy Over Nearly Nothing. *Journal of Neurotherapy*, *10* (2/3), 59-61.

Schoenberger, N. E., Shiflett, S. C., Esty, M. L., Ochs, L., & Matheis, R. J. (2001). Flexyx neurotherapy system in the treatment of traumatic brain injury: An initial evaluation. *Journal of Head Trauma Rehabilitation*, *16* (3), 260-274.

Tansey, M. A. (1990). Righting the rhythms of reason: EEG biofeedback training as a therapeutic modality in a clinical office setting. *Medical Psychotherapy*, *3*, 57-68.

doi:10.1300/J184v10n02_06

Effective Use of LENS Unit as an Adjunct to Cognitive Neuro-Developmental Training

Curtis T. Cripe, PhD

SUMMARY. This article describes three case studies where the Low Energy Neurofeedback System (LENS) was used to augment neurotherapy/neuro-development training to help overcome cognitive and developmental issues. Simultaneously applying neuro-developmental exercises and LENS training has reduced treatment time in our clinic for certain conditions such as Pervasive Developmental Disorder (PDD) and Autistic Spectrum Disorder. The LENS training actually seems responsible for allowing other forms of treatment to take place.

The first case study was of 4 1/2-year-old identical twins, with developmental delay and autistic spectrum that completed their training within 18 months and graduated out of our program symptom-free, performing as normal 6-year-olds. The second case involved Attention Deficit Disorder with hyperactivity and Oppositional Defiant Disorder in a 12-year-old male with comorbid learning and memory issues compounded by undetected food allergies which had affected CNS functioning since birth. The final case was a 43-year-old female with a mild head injury and significant visual and auditory processing problems. In all cases the post-treatment quantitative EEG results demonstrated normalized Z-scores. Cognitive ability testing with the Woodcock-Johnson® III Tests of Cognitive Abilities (Woodcock, McGrew, & Mather, 2001) likewise documented that post-treatment cognitive abilities had normalized. Following the case presentations clinical impressions about LENS training and its effectiveness are presented. doi:10.1300/J184v10n02_07 *[Article copies available for a fee from The Haworth Document Delivery Service: 1-800-HAWORTH. E-mail address: <docdelivery@haworthpress.com> Website: <http://www.HaworthPress.com> © 2006 by The Haworth Press, Inc. All rights reserved.]*

KEYWORDS. Neurotherapy, neuro-development, EEG and cognitive abilities, toxicity

INTRODUCTION

Based on the objectively measured outcomes, we first noticed how effective the addition of the Low Energy Neurofeedback System (LENS) was in working with cases of extreme pervasive developmental disorder (PDD). Later we found it was equally effective in most of the cases coming to our clinic. Due to the nature of the PDD condition, progress can be very slow and in some cases we found these children simply were not able to respond to training without using the LENS treatments. Based on our clinical experience we have found that cases involving excess delta or theta brain wave activity, especially when there is a concurrent underlying medical condition, seem to be particularly responsive to LENS treatment. Assuming that we

Curtis T. Cripe is affiliated with The Crossroads Institute, 18404 North Tatum Boulevard, Suite 207, Phoenix, AZ 85032 (E-mail: ctcripe@att.net).

[Haworth co-indexing entry note]: "Effective Use of LENS Unit as an Adjunct to Cognitive Neuro-Developmental Training." Cripe, Curtis T. Co-published simultaneously in *Journal of Neurotherapy* (The Haworth Medical Press, an imprint of The Haworth Press, Inc.) Vol. 10, No. 2/3, 2006, pp. 79-87; and: *LENS: The Low Energy Neurofeedback System* (ed: D. Corydon Hammond) The Haworth Medical Press, an imprint of The Haworth Press, Inc., 2006, pp. 79-87. Single or multiple copies of this article are available for a fee from The Haworth Document Delivery Service [1-800-HAWORTH, 9:00 a.m. - 5:00 p.m. (EST). E-mail address: docdelivery@haworthpress.com].

address the medical condition and apply a comprehensive neuro-development program which includes LENS training, we make comparable rapid progress with the PDD clients. In our clinical experience we have found LENS treatment is limited or has no effect in cases where there is an excess of beta brain wave activity. We have found that the majority of these cases that involve excess beta activity seem to involve medical conditions, falling under the category of malabsorption and/or neurotoxicity.

Recently in the field of neuroscience, many studies are beginning to demonstrate that cognition, even though it is influenced by genetic factors, is also a developmental age appropriate process based upon the maturation of the client. Specific cognitive abilities are associated with unique EEG patterns in both the non-engaged (resting) and engaged states of different cognitive activities (Goel & Dolan, 2004; Gray, Chabris & Braver, 2003; Prabhakaran, Smith, Desmond, Glover & Gabrieli, 1997; Rivera, Reiss, Eckert & Menon, 2005; Zhang & Poo, 2001). Using quantitative EEG (QEEG) measures along with evoked potentials (EP and ERP) measures, cognitive processes can be quantified and a more specific determination made as to which brain functions appear to be inhibiting an individual's performance (Zani & Proverbio, 2003; Atherton, Zhuang, Bart, Hu, & He, 2003; Aleksandrov, Polyakova, & Stankevich, 2003; Ferstl & von Cramon, 2001; Newman, Carpenter, Varma, & Just, 2003; Geake & Hansen, 2005). When reviewing the biomedical literature it has also been found that some of the underlying cognitive performance problems may be related to underlying health issues which disturb cognitive processes. This results in what can be more accurately described as a loss of functional performance (Beauchaine, 2001; Burgess, Zhang, & Peck, 2000; Porges, 2001; Burns, Baghurst, Sawyer, McMichael, & Tong, 1999; Kidd, 2005; Uhlig, Merkenschlager, Brandmaier, & Egger, 1997; Tang et al., 1999; Eydie et al., 2005). These health/medical issues may include such things as neurotransmitter problems due to mal-absorption issues, allergy irritations, medication effects, etc.

Our clinical assessment procedure evaluates age-appropriate cognitive abilities and performance. This requires us to both understand if the client is functioning at optimal age-appropriate cognitive levels, as well as to understand the underlying reasons why normal performance is not being achieved.

This paper presents three different case studies where LENS was used and where we documented that afterwards functional brain processing issues were normalized. Brain function was measured with both QEEG and psychometric measures of cognitive functioning. The three cases involved (a) developmental issues associated with autistic tendencies, (b) attention deficit disorder (ADD) problems that appeared to be associated with health related issues, and (c) auditory-visual hypersensitivity and learning disability problems associated with a head injury.

METHOD

Analysis Perspective

At the Crossroads Clinic and Centers the focus is on evaluating and improving cognitive abilities. Examining the client from a cognitive neuro-functioning perspective requires one to assess an individual's cognitive abilities as well as to seek to determine the possible root causes of poor cognitive performance. In the educational literature there appear to be four primary schools of thought concerning intellectual cognitive function: (a) the Cattell-Horn-Carroll (CHC) theory (Cattell, 1971; Sternberg, 2000; Sternberg, & Kaufman, 1998; Gilhooly, 1994) which outlines 10 primary cognitive processing domains that interact; (b) the Luria school of thought (Cattell, 1971; Sternberg & Kaufman, 1998; Sternberg, 1998, 2000), which focuses on the interaction between cognitive processing engagement and executive functions; (c) the Gardner school of thought (Gardner, 1983; Sternberg, 2000; Sternberg & Kaufman, 1998) which focuses on cognitive processing styles; and finally (d) the Sternberg method (Sternberg, 2000; Sternberg & Kaufman, 1998) which focuses on the concept of developing life mastery skills. As in personality theory, each school of thought has its place in evaluating a client's overall cognitive profile.

Greenspan and his colleagues (Murray, Clermont, & Brinkley, 2005) defined a term which they called "personal competence," which helps to define many areas of natural cognitive ability. Personal competence is viewed as comprising a set of skills that we use in attaining our goals and solving problems. Cognition refers to the sub-component of these skills involved in thinking and understanding. The Greenspan model consists of three elements: physical competence, personal competence and performance competence.

The evaluation model we use in our clinic model extends the Greenspan model's definition by including a fourth factor adapted from Sternberg's (2000) learned mastery concept. We seek to quantify and track changes in overall levels of performance abilities as a person progresses through our clinic program. This is done through defining in a practical manner what we term PQ™ or Performance Quotient. This initial qualitative mathematical function is defined as: $PQ = w_1*P_1 + w_2*P_2 + w_3*P_3 + w_4*P_4$ and consists of four main weighted (w_i) domains (P_i) with several components: P_1 = physical competence, P_2 = personal competence, P_3 = performance competence, and P_4 = P-factor (the life mastery or maturity level of the child). The broad domains defined above are further divided into twelve sub-domains.

- Physical competence consists of the health of our brain and nervous system, as well as organ (e.g., vision, heart functioning) and motor competence (e.g., strength, coordination).
- Personal competence consists of temperament (e.g., emotionality, distractibility), natural personality (e.g., gregariousness, social orientation), and our level of maturity.
- Performance competence includes practical competence (i.e., the skill to think about and understand problems in everyday settings), conceptual competence (i.e., the skill to think about and understand problems of an academic or abstract nature), language (i.e., the skill to understand and participate in communications), and social competence (i.e., the skill to think about and understand social problems).
- P_i Factor represents both our innate and learned ability to incorporate the concept

of "mastery." It requires that we learn how to interact with life, learn from it, and ultimately contribute to its direction by helping shape the events that come into our world. Generally, this is measured by how we are performing in life.

Weighting factors are determined based upon the initial intake assessment and is biased, based upon the areas where the client needs to focus (i.e., health issues, skill development, development of cognitive abilities). The weighting factor is derived from both objective physiological measures as well as client or parent reports. All P_i factor scores are a combination of physiologic measures, test scores and subjective ratings. Low scores indicate the need for focus on the physiological needs; medium scores suggest the need to focus on personality or skill set development, and higher scores indicate a need for peak performance training or learned mastery skill development. For younger children the importance of using the P_i factor is more apparent than for adults, due to lack of developmentally age appropriate cognitive processing skills which generally are learned at younger ages.

Training Methods

In all cases, training methods included neuro-sensory stimulation during the use of either the LENS unit and/or in combination with conventional neurotherapy. Neuro-sensory stimulation includes tactile, visual, and auditory training, generally targeted towards engagement of frontal/temporal/parietal interactions. More specifically, these consist of a series of exercises uniquely assigned and tailored to the individual's needs. Training exercises and neurotherapy protocols were selected based upon the QEEG, cognitive ERP data, and standardized cognitive performance test data obtained through cognitive ability tests, as well as client goals. As the sessions progressed, exercises and protocols were adjusted during treatment based upon follow-up QEEGs, ERPs, and cognitive performance testing.

Case 1: Autistic Spectrum Disorder

Identical twins entered the program at age 4 1/2. Both girls were cognitively present, but overall age maturation was estimated at only about 24 to 30 months of age based upon the Nepsy (Kirk, Korkman, & Kemp, 1999) and Doman Delacato (Doman, Spitz, Zucman, Delacato, & Doman, 1960) scores. They both fell within the Autistic Spectrum Disorder (ASD) based upon the Gilliam Autism Rating Scale (Gilliam, 2002) and had previously been diagnosed with the classification of ASD. Language expression was "twin speak," in that you could only understand some of their expressions, but they knew what was being said between them. When looking at their QEEGs both girls had nearly identical values within all frequency bands. The most remarkable features included excess absolute delta and beta values, which exceeded three Z-scores as well as hypercoherence in all frequency bands in excess of three Z-scores. Medical measures showed that there was a significant gut dysbiosis (intestinal inflammation often affecting nutritional absorption, due to many possible underlying issues including yeast overgrowth, food allergies, antibiotic reactions, etc.) for both girls, as well as heavy metal in their system. It appeared from other medically based measures that their neuro-immuoendocrine systems were in a hypersensitive state which resulted in other autonomic reactivities.

Looking at the Performance Quotient (PQ) factor it was apparent that treatment bias needed to be toward remediating the physiological system and promoting enhanced cognitive performance, which meant helping them mature to a more age appropriate natural ability. For both girls the more problematic cognitive systems were the auditory memory system, as well as auditory processing, which impacted their overall maturation and ability to engage socially.

Treatment for both girls consisted of a two pronged approach that included a set of sensory integration/differentiation exercises along with a set of cognitive development exercises. This was combined with a medically based set of treatments targeted at improving the function of the gut, organ systems, and replenishing nutritional support which biological test results determined was missing. During each of their treatment sessions neuro-developmental exercises were applied along with targeted auditory training in conjunction with LENS neurofeedback. In working with this population we discovered empirically that during auditory training sessions, if we would apply the LENS training in each session for a certain number of seconds in sequence at electrode sites F4, F3, Fz, Cz, and Pz (which we have labeled the "T-Walk™"), these cognitively compromised children subsequently tend to respond more rapidly to their cognitive developmental exercises. Additionally, we find that the sensory systems tend to begin to "calm down" or normalize at a more rapid rate following the introduction of LENS training.

As the twins matured their PQ scores improved so that by the eighth month we needed to shift the treatment focus to teaching social skill sets. Both girls responded well to the program and at age six they have both improved to the point that they now hit their age appropriate developmental milestones. One became right handed and the other left handed. Additionally, their speech improved to a clear non-compromised speech pattern and all cognitive abilities normalized to that of a typical six-year-old. Due to overdependence on each other, catching up on socialization required the children to be placed in different kindergarten class rooms. Table 1 displays the treatment progress of the twins on various ratings, and Figure 1 presents the QEEG of one of the twins that was done at the beginning and at the completion of treatment. The extreme excesses in absolute and relative power beta, as well as absolute and relative power alpha, are almost entirely normalized. The most extreme beta absolute power excesses were at Fz, Pz, Cz, and T5 in the map

TABLE 1. Progress of Case One in Treatment

Treatment time	PQ Score	GARS	Doman-Delacato Indications
Intake	22	130 Severe	23 to 30 month cognitive development
4 months	33	119 above average	33 to 36 month cognitive development
8 months	42	98 average	46 to 60 month cognitive development
12 months	66	69 very low	60 to age appropriate development
18 months	86	12 none	Age appropriate development

FIGURE 1. Case 1 Pre-/Post-Treatment QEEG

Initial Nx Link QEEG

18-Month Follow-Up

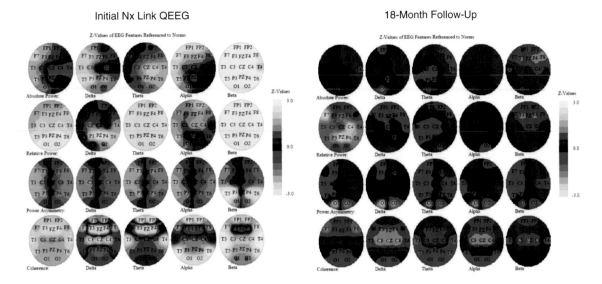

found in Figure 1, and represented deviations of 3.4, 3.1, 3.02, and 2.98 Z-scores, respectively.

Case 2: ADD with Comorbid ODD/Learning and Memory Issues

The second case was a 12-year-old male who was diagnosed by his psychiatrist with Attention Deficit Disorder (ADD) and Oppositional Defiant Disorder (ODD), with comorbid learning and memory problems. Food allergies were discovered to be present which affected central nervous system functioning. The parents believed that this had been a problem since birth. This young man presented clinically as well intended, but extremely absent-minded or inattentive, as well as argumentative. His grades were mostly Ds because of his failure to turn in homework, combined with his C and high D grades on tests. He was in resource (special classes for academic remediation) for math and reading. He was very cranky and resisted any direction unless it was self-initiated. His scores on the Woodcock Johnson showed low normal General Intellectual Ability (GIA) and attention issues, combined with a problem with auditory working memory.

Medication treatment had been recommended, but he reacted negatively to Ritalin, Concerta and Strattera. The Doman-Delacato developmental profile also validated problems with working memory and suggested a lack of brain

system maturation in the ear and eye dominance factor, and in basic mobility factors. This resulted in anxiety and emotional ups and downs.

His PQ factor score indicated that treatment should focus on health, brain developmental factors and basic academics. A three prong treatment approach was initiated. Specific allergy testing was undertaken with the discovery that an allergy to wheat and dust mites both significantly affected his ability to perform on the classic aural digit span for working memory. In digit span testing his capacity ranged from 2 digits to 4 digits. For his age he should have been attaining digits span scores of 6 or more, which he was able to attain after three months of treatment.

LENS neurofeedback was used to help reduce the excessive delta and theta brainwave activity as well as to augment his developmental memory training during lab sessions. During his in-office lab training sessions he performed neuro-developmental exercises along with conventional theta inhibit/SMR enhance neurotherapy protocols based upon his QEEG. The results after 24 sessions showed his performance at school had improved in most classes from Ds to Cs and Cs to B +. At the end of 12 weeks he had graduated out of resource classes, but he was still struggling with his basic reading comprehension.

Initially, the family did not want to address his academic issues, hoping they would just clear up, but his PQ factor indicated a need to shift to enhancing his personal skill sets. The Wide Range Achievement Test III (Wilkinson, 1993) was administered and it was discovered that it would be necessary for the young man to relearn some academic basics in the area of vocabulary building and reading strategies. A tutoring program was recommended and implemented, which allowed his academic test grades in the classroom to catch up. On a personality level, this initially cranky 12-year-old became quite pleasant and helpful to staff. Similar reports by his parents were made on his a six month follow up. Table 2 summarizes treatment progress, and Figure 2 displays his pre- and post-treatment QEEG findings. As seen in Figure 2, the extreme excesses of absolute

power across frequency bands were normalized by the end of six months.

Case 3: Mild Head Injury

The final case is a 43-year-old female who was suffering from a mild head injury with significant visual and auditory processing hypersensitivity. The sensory hypersensitivity created harsh headaches and emotional pain. The accident occurred from a hit-and-run car accident two years prior to her coming to our office. She also presented with problems with memory, focus and attention. Memory aural and visual digit span scores indicated that something was interfering with her memory system interactions. Her General Intellectual Abilities (GIA) score on the Woodcock-Johnson III Test of Cognitive Abilities (Woodcock et al., 2001)

TABLE 2. Progress of Case Two in Treatment

Treatment time	PQ Score	WJC III	Doman-Delacato Indications
Intake	33	GIA 83-89 weak thinking ability, normal cognitive efficiency	Need for memory work, cross pattern
2-months	63	GIA 98-104 normal thinking ability, normal cognitive efficiency	Need for memory work, cross pattern
6-month follow up	88	GIA 105-115 normal thinking ability, normal cognitive efficiency	Within normal ranges

FIGURE 2. Pre-/Post-Treatment QEEGs for Case 2

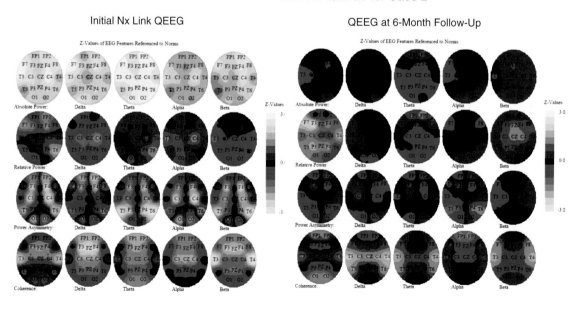

was between 83 and 95, far below her level of educational achievement. (She had a bachelor's degree in English.) Testing on the Doman-Delacato profile indicated that her developmental profile was age appropriate and her lack of cognitive performance was most likely due to a loss of memory function. She was assigned cognitive development exercises which consisted mostly of sensory system desensitization combined with auditory and other cognitive developmental training as indicated by her QEEG and other testing. Within twelve sessions of using the LENS combined with frequency specific auditory training, her hypersensitivity to both sound and light began to normalize as indicated from retesting and her self report. Cognitive function returned to normal within 20 sessions.

Table 3 summarizes her treatment progress and Figure 3 presents her pre-/post-treatment QEEG results. The pre-treatment QEEG showed excess absolute power alpha and in absolute power averaged across frequency bands. This was no longer present after treatment. The patient's traumatic brain injury discriminant function scores and patterns normalized following treatment.

DISCUSSION AND CONCLUSION

Neurotherapy with the LENS is one of many tools that we use. It has been our experience that LENS can be very effective when used appropriately and in conjunction with neurodevelopment, bio-chemical, physiological and body health interventions. The LENS unit acts as a very precise and specific tool. It is my impression, as was the case with the twins cited above, that patients who are more significantly developmentally and learning disabled, or individuals with brain injuries are able to progress in neurocognitive exercises because of the facilitating effects that come from LENS training. Commonly LENS training seems to help jump start cognitive systems, as it did with the twins, and not only allow them to perceive what is being asked of them, but also allow them to be able to engage in the neuro-rehabilitation exercises. In the case of the 12-year-old ADD/ODD male cited in this paper, LENS training seemed to not only accelerate the progress of this young man, but it also enabled us to help normalize the auditory processing to allow more normal auditory perceptual integration. For the 43-year-old woman who had experienced a traumatic head injury, the LENS unit affected a change in her hypersensitivity to both the auditory and visual input. The LENS training seemed to be the factor that allowed subsequent desensitization exercises to become more effective, reducing treatment time, and allowing her to regain normal functioning of her auditory and visual brain systems.

Although our clinical results are uncontrolled and confounded by the inclusion of other forms of treatment, it was our experience that prior to implementing LENS training our treatment program with both children and adults required 8 to 12 months for us to achieve the same results that we are now achieving within 3 to 6 months, once we added the component of LENS training. It appears that LENS neurofeedback may be able to help accelerate the reduction of the slow brainwave activity during our treatment of allergies, as well as help augment the performance of the memory exercises during neurocognitive training sessions.

TABLE 3. Summary of Treatment Progress in Case 3

Treatment time	PQ Score	WJC III	Doman-Delacato Indications
Intake	55	GIA 83-95 (weak thinking ability, weak cognitive efficiency)	Normal development, hypersensitive sensory processing
2-months	83	GIA 110-115 (normal range thinking ability, normal cognitive efficiency)	Normal development, sensitive sensory processing
6-month Follow up	93	GIA 110-115 (normal thinking ability, normal cognitive efficiency)	Normal development, normal sensory processing

FIGURE 3. Pre-/Post-Treatment QEEGs and Brain Injury Discriminant Scores

Initial NxLink and Neuroguide Mild Traumatic Brain Injury Discriminate Match

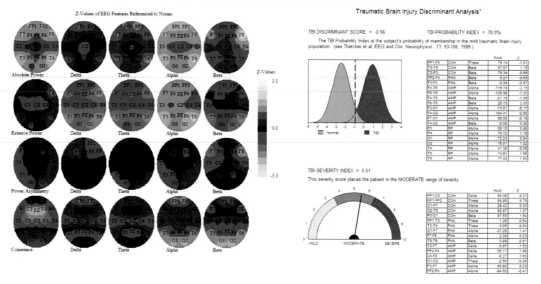

6-Month Follow-Up

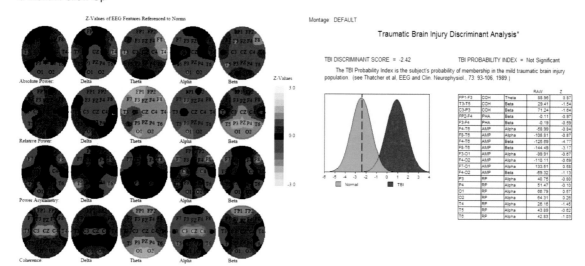

REFERENCES

Aleksandrov, A. A., Polyakova, N. V., & Stankevich, L. N. (2003). Evoked brain potentials in adolescents in normal conditions and in attention deficit during solution of tasks requiring recognition of short-duration acoustic stimuli. *Neuroscience & Behavioral Physiology*, 35 (2), 153-157.

Atherton, M., Zhuang, J., Bart, W. M., Hu, X., & He, S. (2003). A functional MRI study of high-level cognition. I. The game of chess. *Brain Research & Cognitive Brain Research*, 16 (1), 26-31.

Beauchaine, T. (2001). Vagal tone, development, and Gray's motivational theory: Toward an integrated model of autonomic nervous system functioning in psychopathology. *Development and Psychopathology*, 13, 183-214.

Burgess, J. R., Stevens, L., Zhang, W., & Peck, L. (2000). Long-chain polyunsaturated fatty acids in children with attention-deficit hyperactivity disorder. *American Journal of Clinical Nutrition*, 711 (Suppl.), 323-327.

Burns, J. M., Baghurst, P. A., Sawyer, M. G., McMichael, A. J., & Tong, S. L. (1999). Lifetime low-level exposure to environmental lead and children's emotional and behavioral development at ages 11-13 years. The Port Pirie Cohort Study. *American Journal of Epidemiology, 149* (8), 740-749.

Cattell, R. B. (1971). *Abilities: Their structure, growth and action.* Boston: Houghton-Mifflin.

Doman, R. J., Spitz, E. R., Zucman, E., Delacato, C. H., & Doman, G. (1960). Children with severe brain injuries: Neurological organization in terms of mobility. *Journal of the American Medical Association, 174,* 257-262.

Eydie L. Kolko, M., Bogen, D., Perel, J., Bregar, A., Uhl, K., et al. (2005). Neonatal signs after late in utero exposure to serotonin reuptake inhibitors. *Journal of the American Medical Association, 293,* 2372-2383.

Ferstl, E. C., & von Cramon, D. Y. (2001). The role of coherence and cohesion in text comprehension: An event-related fMRI study. *Brain Research & Cognitive Brain Research, 11* (3), 325-340.

Gardner, H. (1983). *Frames of mind: The theory of multiple intelligences.* New York: Basic Books.

Geake, J. G., & Hansen, P. C. (2005). Neural correlates of intelligence as revealed by fMRI of fluid analogies. *Neuroimage, 26* (2), 555-564.

Gilhooly, K. J. (1994). Knowledge. In R.J. Sternberg (Ed.), *Encyclopedia of human intelligence* (pp. 636-638). New York: Macmillan.

Gilliam, J. E. (2002). *Autism rating scales.* Circle Pines, MN: AGS Press.

Goel, V., & Dolan, R. J. (2004). Differential involvement of left prefrontal cortex in inductive and deductive reasoning. *Cognition, 93* (3), 109-121.

Gray, J. R., Chabris, C. F., & Braver, T. S. (2003). Neural mechanisms of general fluid intelligence. *Nature Neuroscience, 6* (3), 316-322.

Kidd, P. M. (2005). Neurodegeneration from mitochondrial insufficiency: nutrients, stem cells, growth factors, and prospects for brain rebuilding using integrative management. *Alternative Medicine Review, 10* (4), 268-293.

Kirk, U., Korkman, M., & Kemp, S. (1999). *Essentials of NEPSY assessment.* New York-Chichester: Wiley.

Murray, T. S., Clermont, Y., & Binkley, M. (2005). International Adult Literacy Survey Measuring Adult Literacy and Life Skills. Ottawa: New Frameworks Catalogue no. 89-552-MIE, no. 13.

Newman, S. D., Carpenter, P. A., Varma, S., & Just, M. A. (2003). Frontal and parietal participation in problem solving in the Tower of London: fMRI and computational modeling of planning and high-level perception. *Neuropsychologia, 41* (12), 1668-1682.

Porges, S. W. (2001). The polyvagal theory: phylogenetic substrates of a social nervous system. *International Journal of Psychophysiology, 42,* 123-146.

Prabhakaran, V., Smith, J. A., Desmond, J. E., Glover, G. H., & Gabrieli, J. D. (1997). Neural substrates of fluid reasoning: an fMRI study of neocortical activation during performance of the Raven's Progressive Matrices Test. *Cognitive Psychology, 33* (1), 43-63.

Rivera, S. M., Reiss, A. L., Eckert, M. A., & Menon, V. (2005). Developmental changes in mental arithmetic: Evidence for increased functional specialization in the left inferior parietal cortex. *Cerebral Cortex, 15* (11), 1779-1790.

Sternberg, R. J. (1998). Abilities are forms of developing expertise. *Educational Researcher, 27* (3), 11-20.

Sternberg, R. J. (2000). *Handbook of intelligence.* New York: Cambridge.

Sternberg, R. J., & Kaufman, J. C. (1998). Human abilities. *Annual Review of Psychology, 49,* 1134-1139.

Tang, H. W., Huel, G., Campagna, D., Hellier, G., Boissinot, C., & Blot, P. (1999). Neurodevelopmental evaluation of 9-month-old infants exposed to low levels of lead in utero: involvement of monoamine neurotransmitters. *Journal of Applied Toxicology, 19* (3), 167-72.

Uhlig, T., Merkenschlager, A., Brandmaier, R., & Egger, J. (1997). Topographic mapping of brain electrical activity in children with food-induced attention deficit hyperkinetic disorder. *European Journal of Pediatrics, 6* (7), 557-561.

Wilkinson, G. S. (1993). *Wide Range Achievement Test-III. Administration Manual.* Wilmington, DE: Wide Range, Inc.

Woodcock, R. W., McGrew, K. S., & Mather, N. (2001). Essentials of Woodcock-Johnson III Cognitive Abilities Assessment. Itasca, IL: Riverside Publishing.

Zani, A., & Proverbio, A. M. (2003). *The cognitive electrophysiology of mind and brain.* New York: Academic Press.

Zhang, L. I., & Poo, M. (2001). Electrical activity and development of neural circuits. *Nature Neuroscience, 4,* 1207-1214.

doi:10.1300/J184v10n02_07

The LENS Neurofeedback with Animals

Stephen Larsen, PhD
Robin Larsen, PhD
D. Corydon Hammond, PhD
Stephen Sheppard, PhD
Len Ochs, PhD
Sloan Johnson, MA
Carla Adinaro, ARIA-Cert
Carrie Chapman, BA

SUMMARY. *Background.* A customary route for research in the life sciences is to begin with animal studies, and only after thorough evaluation, attempt the same procedure with humans. In this pilot clinical outcomes study, the inverse procedure is followed. Encouraging results in the areas of CNS regulation led clinicians to explore whether the method is equally effective with animals who suffered the same problems as humans. The qualities studied included aggressiveness, mood instability, hypervigilance, inability to learn from experience. Species studies over about three years consisted of horses, dogs, and cats.

Method. All animals were treated on the Low Energy Neurofeedback System (LENS) using the I-330 C2, the mini-C2, or the GP plus EEG processor with a laptop computer. Unlike with human subjects, it was impossible to use "eyes-closed" condition, so blink artifact was impossible to rule out. Animals stood in stalls, tied to hitching posts (horses), or on the floor or in their owner's lap (dogs and cats). With most animals the "stim" condition was used, with a brief second or two of stimulation embedded in a longer period of "no-stim," four to twenty seconds depending on the situation. Where possible, a cortical map was done of from ten to twelve sites on the animal version of the standardized mapping system developed by Holliday and Williams (1999, 2003) to match human mapping. Since it has become available several months ago, the Animal CNS Questionnaire was used, and a five symptom or more "Subjective Symptom Checklist" completed on each treatment session with the owner. Narrative reports were collected from owners, but also from professional animal trainers and handlers. In some cases animals were photographed or videotaped before and after.

Results. The animal studies are similar in outcome to the human results. As judged by owners, independent witnesses and professional trainers and handlers, animal behavior improves in the di-

Stephen Larsen is Psychology Professor Emeritus at SUNY, Ulster, and Director of the Stone Mountain Center.

Robin Larsen, Carla Adinaro, and Carrie Chapman are affiliated with the Stone Mountain Center.

D. Corydon Hammond is Professor, Physical Medicine and Rehabilitation, University of Utah School of Medicine.

Stephen Sheppard is affiliated with the University of Utah School of Medicine.

Len Ochs is affiliated with Ochs Labs, Sebastopol, CA.

Sloan Johnson is in private practice in Mill Valley, CA.

Address correspondence to: Stephen Larsen, 310 River Road Extension, New Paltz, NY 12561 (E-mail: office@stonemountaincenter.com).

[Haworth co-indexing entry note]: "The LENS Neurofeedback with Animals." Larsen, Stephen et al. Co-published simultaneously in *Journal of Neurotherapy* (The Haworth Medical Press, an imprint of The Haworth Press, Inc.) Vol. 10, No. 2/3, 2006, pp. 89-104; and: *LENS: The Low Energy Neurofeedback System* (ed: D. Corydon Hammond) The Haworth Medical Press, an imprint of The Haworth Press, Inc., 2006, pp. 89-104. Single or multiple copies of this article are available for a fee from The Haworth Document Delivery Service [1-800-HAWORTH, 9:00 a.m. - 5:00 p.m. (EST). E-mail address: docdelivery@haworthpress.com].

mensions of flexibility, calmness, emotional stability, intelligence and problem solving The authors did not feel placebo "controls" were necessary or appropriate to these experiments. They had head injuries, survived natural catastrophes, or were abused or neglected (sorry to say) by owners. What was observed, in case after case, is that the more treatments administered the "easier" it became to administer additional treatments (animals were more complaint and calm).

Conclusion/Discussion. Results with animals are parallel to and confirmatory of results with human children and adults. Animals may be traumatized by many causes, not the least of which are human in origin. Thus it is rewarding to see a human procedure help them. With treatment, the animals seem more calm, adaptable, and natural. Some of the results resemble the easy and short-term treatments of human children and infants, who have not yet had a chance to acquire (more difficult to dislodge) habits and defense mechanisms around their problems. These studies are highly preliminary, but very encouraging. The authors would love to see the LENS method applied to a variety of species and in ever-increasing numbers. doi:10.1300/J184v10n02_08 *[Article copies available for a fee from The Haworth Document Delivery Service: 1-800-HAWORTH. E-mail address: <docdelivery@ haworthpress.com> Website: <http://www.HaworthPress.com> © 2006 by The Haworth Press, Inc. All rights reserved.]*

KEYWORDS. Neurofeedback, EEG biofeedback, veterinary, behavior modification, animal behavior, animal training, animal EEG

INTRODUCTION

In the life sciences animal research has led to the discovery of many useful things with applicability to human health, illness, and its treatment. During the 1960s Neal Miller (1969), at Rockefeller University, was studying pleasure-center brain stimulation on rats paralyzed by curare. In response to a reinforcing stimulation the rats were able to speed or slow their heartbeat without muscular movement of any kind. Miller's work paralleled the work of Green, Green and Walters (1970) and Green and Green (1986) with yogis that showed that humans could likewise speed and slow their heart rate through meditative techniques.

Sterman and Friar (1971) and Sterman (1977), pioneers in the field of neurofeedback, discovered that brainwave patterns in cats could be modified and trained by operant conditioning. Cats that were able to increase the sensorimotor rhythm (SMR) were discovered to become much more seizure-resistant when they were later exposed to a toxic chemical that caused seizures. This serendipitous discovery led to research that successfully documented the ability of neurofeedback to reduce seizures in humans who suffered with uncontrolled epilepsy (Sterman & Friar, 2000; Egner & Sterman, 2006).

Thus Sterman's animal research with cats provided the foundation for assisting epilepsy patients, including workers in the aerospace industry who had been exposed to the toxic effects of monomethylhydrazine, a volatile component of rocket fuels. Sterman's discoveries initiated a whole generation of brainwave researchers exploring the potentials of neurofeedback with ADD/ADHD (Lubar, 2003; Monastra et al., 2005) and in a variety of other areas (Hammond, in press) including alcoholism and post-traumatic stress disorder (Peniston & Kulkosky, 1991; Peniston, Marrinan, Deming, & Kulkosky, 1993), learning disabilities (Fernandez et al., 2003), peak performance training (Egner & Gruzelier, 2003; Raymond, Sajid, Parkinson, & Gruzelier, 2005), and anxiety and depression (Hammond, 2005; Moore, 2000). Margaret Ayers, who uses a system with digital real-time neurofeedback, has also indicated that she has successfully treated dogs and horses with neurofeedback in the past twenty years (Ayers, 1987; Ayers, M. A., personal communication, September 10, 2005).

However, apart from Sterman's research and some unpublished case reports of Margaret Ayers, neurotherapy has only been applied to humans. This paper will report on the use of the Low Energy Neurofeedback System (LENS) in the treatment of a variety of problems in animals.

The LENS (Ochs, 2006) provides a unique and passive form of neurofeedback which produces its effects through the introduction of a very tiny electromagnetic signal. This stimulation, which is far weaker than the input we receive from simply holding a cell phone to our ear, is delivered for one second at a time down electrode wires. The frequency of the electromagnetic stimulation is determined, moment-to-moment, by the dominant frequency of the EEG which is measured in hertz or cycles per second, and updated 16 times per second. The client sits eyes closed, and the total time in which electromagnetic fields are received in a treatment session is usually only a few seconds at a small number of electrode sites on the head. This stimulation is believed to gently nudge the brain off of its stuck points, assisting it to become more flexible and self-regulating. Research (e.g., Donaldson, Sella, & Mueller, 1998; Mueller, Donaldson, Nelson, & Layman, 2001; Larsen, 2006; Schoenberger, Shiflett, Esty, Ochs, & Matheis, 2001), as well as clinical experience has found LENS rivals traditional forms of neurofeedback in the treatment of conditions such as traumatic brain injury, fibromyalgia, ADD/ADHD, depression, and other conditions (Larsen, 2006; Ochs, 1994, 1996).

As shown in the CNS Questionnaire for Animals (see Appendix), animals often suffer from some of the same brain and CNS-based problems as humans: epilepsy, brain injuries, aggressiveness, depression, anxiety, lethargy, clumsiness, hypervigilance, restlessness, and attentional problems. Encouraged by the positive results with LENS training in humans, in 2003 we began to see if the LENS would assist in remediating problems in animals. The cases presented in this paper were collected from several different clinicians over about two and a half years. There are also some comments from Carla Adinaro, a professional dressage trainer, and other animal handlers. Other cases on the use of LENS with animals have been reported in an earlier publication (Larsen, 2006). We will summarize a few of the early cases from Larsen (2006) and then proceed in reporting some new cases in more detail.

METHOD

Animals were sometimes evaluated with a LENS map (Ochs, 2006) utilizing the veteri-nary version of the International 10-20 system of electrode placement, as published in Holliday and Williams (1999) and displayed in Figure 1. It can be seen that although the site map is depicted on a horse's brain, the same quantitative LENS mapping analysis procedures that are used in humans can be used in doing animal analyses. This was found to be appropriate in the cases where mapping was done, as if the difference between animals and humans were less important than the similarities. In general, the same brain wave ranges, as measured in hertz, and the same meanings attributed to high amplitude waves (measured in microvolts) seemed to be observed. All mapping and treatments were done with the J&J Engineering I-330 C2 and mini-C2 hardware.

Where it was not possible to do mapping, but treatment was urgent and the animal too aggressive to allow mapping, C3 and C4 electrode sites were used in treatment. This was especially true in cats and in small dogs where the heads are so small that it is difficult to differen-

FIGURE 1. Equine EEG (Adapted from Holliday and Williams, 1999)

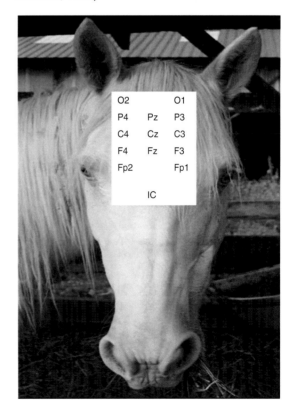

tiate where one site left off and another began, especially when our standard size electrodes were used with very small animals. Although clinical experience (Ochs, 2006) has found that treatment in humans that is guided by a LENS mapping assessment is more effective, thus far we have no observations or data evaluating the efficacy of using mapping procedures to guide treatment in animals, versus using a more generic treatment approach using only C3 and C4 electrode sites.

Even though animals might be as sensitive or reactive as humans, in all the cases studied in this paper, the "stim" condition (10-18 Watts per sq.cm.) was used, while the energy background of the equipment was the "lo-stim" (10-21Watts per sq.cm.) as discussed by Ochs (2006). Two to six seconds of total treatment was the most commonly used protocol. The only mild over-stimulation effect that was observed in one case was when a clinician gave several seconds of treatment at each of five sites. The owner reported that the horse seemed "dopey" and somewhat clumsy the next day. As we commonly find with humans, the over-stimulation side effect wore off after about twenty-four hours and the horse showed behavioral improvement thereafter.

Treatment results with animals were evaluated by changes in behavior, body language, expression, energy, adaptability, and flexibility. Systematic symptom ratings were obtained on a number of the animals.

RESULTS

We will first briefly review several cases and then present the results of two recent cases.

Moondog

The very first animal we studied was "Moondog," a thirteen-year-old "Aussie" or Australian Shepherd, owned by Stephen and Robin Larsen, who showed depression and dyspraxia, possibly following a stroke and a series of spinal injuries that resulted from being struck by thousand-pound horses as she valiantly tried to "herd" them. Prior to treatment she was subdued and walked awkwardly with her back legs not "tracking" with her front legs. Felicitously,

her treatment occurred during a LENS training program for professionals, and her condition before and afterwards were observed by a number of trained clinicians and skilled animal handlers.

Following treatment Moondog was noticeably more "perky," acting less depressed in her body language. Her sense of curiosity seemed to return and she explored her environment more actively. Her back legs became coordinated with her front legs. She was less clumsy and could climb in and out of cars better and ascend steps with more ease. Treatment was continued over her last two years of life at a frequency of about once a month. Moondog passed away in August, 2004 at almost 15 years of age. Moondog can be seen in Figure 2.

Dutch

Our next, quite exciting, animal case was Dutch, a "killer" horse who had been badly abused and would strike out at handlers with his hooves or pin people against walls. Adrenalin, and the idea of treating a horse with an evil reputation in a gloomy, unlit barn, did not keep us from observing dramatic changes in the horse's body language, after only two seconds of treatment each at C3 and at C4. These nonverbal changes included a huge sigh, a lowering of the head, and the commencing of a chewing response (indicating parasympathetic as opposed to sympathetic nervous system dominance). Dutch, who is seen in Figure 3, only received one treatment, but his owner/rescuer said he was more easily managed afterwards.

Dizzy

Dizzy the cat was our first feline subject (also seen in Figure 2). Though large and formidable

FIGURE 2. Moondog and Dizzy

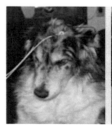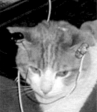

FIGURE 3. Dutch, the "Killer" Horse

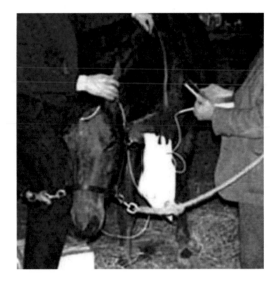

looking, he knew he was the "outsider" (owned by a woman staying for a few months in our guest house). Our own house cats, though smaller, had their home territory well established. Mother and daughter, they would gang up on the hapless Dizzy and terrorize him day or night. He presented as being hypervigilant and extremely anxious. His owner said he was fearful and wary most of the time.

Dizzy was held while the electrodes and paste were applied (Dizzy loved the electrodes and paste). A thick towel was placed on the lap of the person holding Dizzy during the treatment so she would not get little puncture wounds in her leg. During the LENS procedure our two house cats came around, full of indignation that this interloper was being entertained in the living room. They sat on the other side of a plate glass window and glared in the direction of the terrified and agitated Dizzy, while growling in stereo. Their attentions helped to distract Dizzy from the treatment procedure, however, and he received only 1 second of stimulation at C3 and 1 second at C4 (at a 20 Hz offset). After being released, he fled into the woodpile at high speed, only once looking back with a look that seemed to say, "All humans are definitely crazy."

It was not until two days later that one of the experimenters saw a strange thing. Arlecchina, one of the house cats, was growling, hissing loudly and slowly backing up along the porch, clearly nonplussed by a menacing *something*.

Expecting to see a dog or even a fox, we were completely astonished by the stealthy advance of Dizzy toward his former adversary, somehow miraculously reversing the roles. Thereafter, over about three weeks until Dizzy and his owner departed, he held his ground and gave a little better than he got back to his tormentors.

Silver

Silver (see Figure 4) was an abused horse that came to the Stone Mountain Farm four years ago, at about fourteen years of age. He often seemed wary and grumpy. An albino Appaloosa, he was very myopic and light-sensitive. He was dyspraxic and tended to stumble when ridden. When being trained, or longed (trained on a line), he was mistrustful and short-tempered. While being groomed he would nip at people, grabbing their clothes or flesh–a response seldom found in a happy and balanced horse.

We were able to perform a LENS topographic map on Silver, which (as seen in Figure 4) revealed a very high-amplitude, dysregulated right frontal area (probably associated with an injury). After the mapping and a few stim treatments of no more than four seconds per treatment, our dressage instructor noticed that his expression had changed. Quite a number of people remarked that he seemed friendlier and happier. He no longer nipped at people.

Not long after treatment Silver was moved to a different farm. A horse trainer began to work with him and found him responsive and able to learn. He is being ridden as a trail horse and stumbles much less. He is now known as a "ridable" horse.

More Recent Cases

Gandalf the Grey (a rescued dog). Gandalf is a purebred Australian Shepherd dog. This breed (like Moondog) is known for their intelligence, vigilance, social instincts, and desire to herd everything from sheep to SUVs. Gandalf was purchased from a pet store, but his owners found him too active and energetic, so he spent nine months of his first year mostly in a "crate." Neighbors noticed that the dog was being neglected, because they never saw him in the yard or taken for a walk. After a period of time "Aus-

FIGURE 4. Silver the Horse and His LENS Map

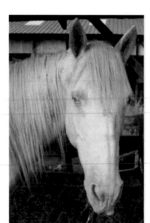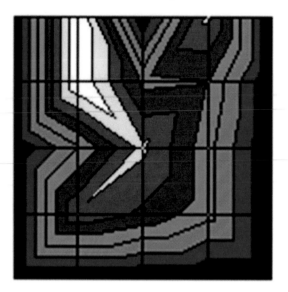

sie Rescue" was called and the dog was brought to an interim home with other dogs. After an interview and site visit, the excellent rescue team agreed to place him with two of the authors at Stone Mountain Farm.

Gandalf was anxious, immature, hypervigilant, extremely noisy, occasionally did fear biting, and was fearful of strangers. He was especially reactive to dark and bearded men (we know nothing of the history that led to this response). He bit a couple of our staff and friends. When we brought him home he was incontinent, erratic, suspicious, and would furiously bark at invisible things. He could not go up and down stairs because of an atrophied back end (from being locked in a cage for so long). The veterinarian said that he had hip dysplasia. He was impulsive, which would be manifested by running away off the leash and car-chasing, as well as "counter-surfing" (we found that many things, supposedly placed out of reach, had a way of disappearing). From his response to the Animal CNS Questionnaire we identified and scored eight areas of concern on a scale from 10 (worst) to zero (no problem). His greatest pre-treatment problems were summarized as hypervigilance (which was manifested by wild barking at most people), anxiety, having a weak back end, impulsiveness, incontinence, social immaturity, "counter surfing," and chasing cars or tractors (or almost anything else). His

average behavior problem ratings before commencing with LENS treatment were 8.75. There was, of course, some overlap between the rated areas. Problem behaviors were rated by staff and others who came in contact with the dog.

Admittedly, treating such an animal was a tricky situation. The Aussie Rescue staff was worried that we would not be able to keep the dog because of his erratic behaviors and that we would have to return him. Gandalf was, of course, also handled gently, but firmly, petted, talked to, taken for rides in the car, fed and exercised, and taken for walks around the farm. Thus these are confounding variables and it is impossible to separate the effects of these ordinary activities with an adopted pet that had been very neglected and damaged, from the neurofeedback. Therefore, neurofeedback can be considered as one (unusual) component in a therapeutic milieu. The LENS treatments followed the map and site sort, averaging two or three sites per treatment, with one second of input at each site. He was given five photonic stimulation treatments of about five minutes each for his hind-end weakness. Photonic stimulation involves the use of infrared light that is used to assist with conditions such as pain, muscle and nerve problems.

The first treatment with Gandalf was extremely difficult because of restlessness, biting at the wires and head-jerking. One treatment with one second of stimulation at C3 and C4 was done before doing a LENS map. Gandalf was held while the electrodes were applied and the computer ran. His shrill barking at the therapy center made the staff and everyone else very jumpy and irritated. We had trepidations about doing a map, but we wanted to guide treatment in the manner that we do with hu-

mans, as well as for research purposes. Mapping was done at 9 sites instead of 13, although Holliday and Williams (1999) advise that it is possible to use 13 electrode sites with a large dog. Gandalf's head was small and thus we decided to stay with the "inner circle" as displayed in Gandalf's maps in Figure 5. The electrode sites we mapped and treated were F3, C3, P3, P4, C4, F4, Fz, Cz, Pz.

FIGURE 5. Gandalf Pre-Treatment LENS Map

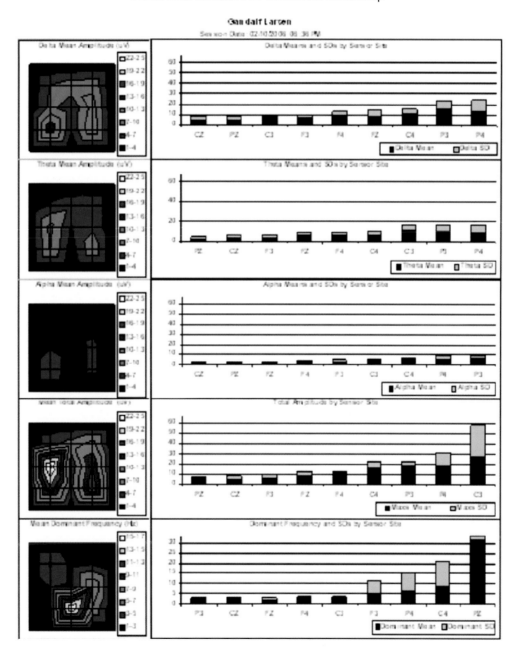

Photonic stimulation treatment was extremely difficult. Gandalf seemed to think the photon stimulator or its wand were a kind of sinister vacuum cleaner, intent on making him miserable. However, with this treatment too, he learned to stand still and receive it after the first few treatments. The post treatment results can be seen in Figure 6 which shows the Gandalf Lens Map indicating low amplitudes and decrease in bright colors on the histogram.

As of the time of the second ratings there is no doubt about his new family keeping Gandalf the Grey. As the anxiety has relaxed, a loving and cute doggy nature has come out. He is far more playful. He has become a champion ball and Frisbee chaser. If left in the car while we are shopping or in a restaurant, he waits patiently. He has bonded with several of our most frequently seen dark-bearded male patients, and

FIGURE 6. Gandalf Post-Treatment LENS Map

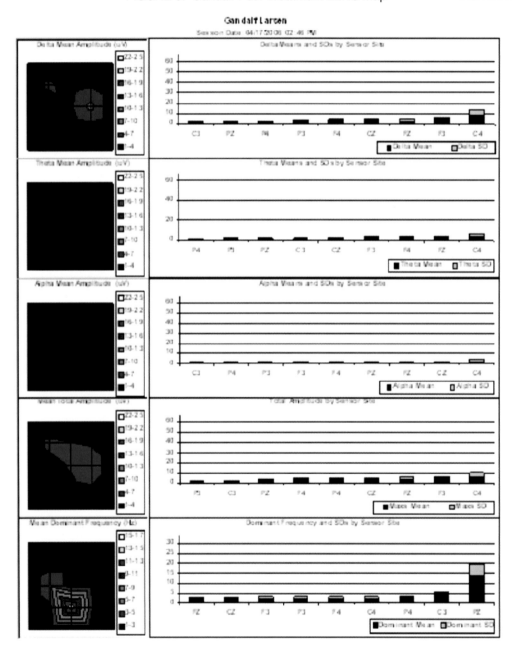

no longer barks hysterically at them–in fact, he cuddles nicely with one bearded gentleman. He was initially guarded and aversive toward a bearded male who was wearing a large felt hat when Gandalf first met him. He barked and growled incessantly and shrilly. Now he follows the same man around, responds to commands of "sit" and "down," lying all the way down, and occasionally coming over and resting his head on the man's knee while seeming to smile a doggy smile.

Jock the Dog. Jock was an English Bull Terrier, born in July of 2004. His owners acquired him at eight weeks of age from a breeder in South Africa. He seemed quite normal for the first five to six months of his life. He was very playful, affectionate, and trainable. He was given a lot of activity including frequent hikes in the mountains and plenty of off-leash exercise each week at a local nature park. He graduated from a six-week puppy obedience class and a six-week basic obedience class. He did not have any problems with house training or separation anxiety. He could be described as "headstrong," but at a normal level for bull terriers.

At about five to six months of age, Jock began chasing his tail and even biting his tail when he could catch it. This was fairly infrequent at first, but gradually became a very frequent behavior. Although he had a very active lifestyle, it was speculated that he perhaps needed even more activity and the frequency of his exercise was increased from three to four times per week to almost daily. That seemed to help for a while. It was also noted that defecating seemed to help to some degree.

Unfortunately, Jock's tail chasing gradually became more frequent, of longer duration, and more intense. By fifteen months of age, he was spending between 30 and 50 percent of his waking time chasing his tail. He even began interrupting favorite activities such as playing and hiking to chase his tail. It also became increasingly difficult to distract him from this activity.

The concerns of his owners that his tail chasing might be related to an emotional problem increased, but this was eventually ruled out by a veterinarian. He was placed on Amitryptaline, but this did not improve his behavior. One of his owners works seasonally and was able to spend time with him most of the day every day, pro-

viding him with a great deal of attention, affection, and playtime. As a result, boredom and loneliness could be ruled out. He was generally very well-behaved and rarely needed to be disciplined. His owners tried a variety of behavioral interventions to address the tail chasing, such as interrupting the behavior and rewarding alternative behaviors, but this did not help. Jock was also very sociable and got along very well with people and other dogs. These factors convinced his owners that his tail chasing had a medical basis.

Finally, Jock began to experience personality changes. As noted, he was generally very sociable and not in the least aggressive. However, he began showing increased irritability at night. This first began at about one year of age and was most consistent in the evenings. For example, if he fell asleep in the evening before his normal bedtime and was then awakened, he would become irritable and growl. His hair would stand up and he would walk about with very stiff legs. This went on for several months. He had a one-week episode of snapping at his owner's feet when awakened, but this subsided. However, at about fifteen months of age he attacked and bit his owner's ankle without warning. This occurred in the morning and he continued to have outbursts of aggression for several hours thereafter. At the same time, his legs were noted to shake fairly vigorously. This was very unusual behavior, especially given that the morning was one of his most affectionate times of the day. From that point on, he displayed violent aggression if awakened suddenly in the morning or in the evening. He was usually good natured during the day, but continued to have progressive problems with tail-chasing. His owners attempted to manage his aggression by kenneling him in the evening and gradually waking him up in the morning. This primarily prevented violent outbursts, but he continued to show irritability and growling.

The tail chasing combined with the personality changes and violent outbursts convinced his owners that something of a medical nature was wrong. He received progressively increased attention from veterinarians, particularly after the violent outbursts. This included a veterinarian with a 30-year history of breeding bull terriers and consultation from specialists at Tufts University School of Veterinary Science. Jock's blood chemistry (including thyroid function) was normal. Blood tests indicated normal kidney and liver function. A hypo-allergenic diet was tried, but without benefit. Ultimately, the aggression and tail-chasing were diagnosed as being due to a complex partial seizure disorder. The tail chasing syndrome is not well understood, but it is being actively researched from a genetic standpoint at Tufts University. There has been some speculation that this is a form of predatory behavior that is essentially "misfiring" and associated with seizure activity. The violence problems were described as a "rage syndrome," most common in cocker spaniels. Like Jock, the violent outbursts are most common in cocker spaniels when suddenly going from sleep to wakefulness, but can happen at any time. At about seventeen months of age, Jock bit his owner again, but this time in the face. The bite was severe enough to necessitate twelve stitches. At that point, his owners were on the verge of having Jock euthanized.

In a last ditch attempt to treat Jock's problems, LENS was used. Behavioral ratings for tail chasing, aggression, and other behaviors were started three days prior to Jock's first treatment. It was initially quite difficult to treat Jock with the LENS system. He appeared to be frightened by having electrodes applied to his scalp and ears, and reacted with aggression and strong efforts to escape the situation. Jock was almost 60 pounds of muscle and had been known to pull one of his owners for two miles uphill on cross country skis. Thus, when Jock became aggressive, it was exceptionally difficult to control him. The first attempt at treatment was aborted for these reasons. His veterinarian subsequently prescribed Valium to calm him for each treatment. Jock had a very strong constitution and it required 35mg of Valium to relax him sufficiently to allow the electrodes to be placed and the treatment administered. The initial treatment took place at the clinician's home. However, the novelty of this environment was very stimulating and it was difficult to get Jock to sit still for the procedure, even with the Valium. The first treatment was successfully applied, however, on December 17, 2005. This involved a one-second input each at C3 and C4 locations. It was also found that treating him in his own home environment was much easier. Jock underwent three more treatments at

home on December 18, 23 and 26, 2005. The second and third treatments involved two, one-second inputs to both C3 and C4. The fourth treatment involved a one-second input to C3 and C4.

After the first LENS treatment there was an immediate, dramatic decrease in both tail chasing and irritability. He became much more contented and playful. He engaged in minimal tail chasing and it was easy to redirect him when he did chase his tail. He did not show any aggressiveness in the evening through either growling or outright violence. He continued to essentially sustain these improvements for several days after the second treatment. His personality was very much like it had been prior to the onset of the problems with irritability and aggression. He then began to show a slight increase in nighttime irritability and a more significant increase in tail chasing. His aggression again decreased very dramatically after the third treatment and he essentially had no problems with irritability or aggression from that point onward. The results were really quite startling.

Unfortunately, the tail chasing continued to worsen even after treatments three and four. It reached a point where he was chasing his tail almost continuously when awake. He twice caught and bit his tail to the point of severe bleeding, afterwards thrashing his tail around, flipping blood everywhere throughout the kitchen until it appeared like a crime scene. He was chasing his tail so much that he would collapse from exhaustion for a few minutes and then resume this activity. He panted constantly and seemed to be overheating. It was impossible to interrupt his behavior except by holding him. He would whine and shake when held and immediately resume tail chasing when released. Jock seemed to be suffering terribly and was euthanized on December 28, 2005.

It appears that the LENS treatment had a very significant, beneficial impact on Jock's rage problem and presumably his seizures. He reverted to his usual loving, affectionate self almost immediately after the first two treatments. The second through fourth treatments seemed to only reinforce this improvement and his aggression was essentially eliminated. Unfortunately, the LENS treatment only had a temporary benefit with the tail chasing. It is unclear why this was the case. It may be that Jock had a particularly strong genetic basis for this behavior that could not be overcome by the LENS treatment. Alternatively, it may be that the LENS treatment helped the aggression, but perhaps exacerbated the tail chasing, or that treatment at other electrode sites might have provided additional benefits if it had been done. Further research will be needed to investigate the effects of LENS on epileptiform and aggressive behavior. A summary of daily behavioral ratings may be found in Figure 7. It can be seen that following the initial two day baseline, problematic behaviors dramatically decreased and stabilized, with the exception of tail chasing.

DISCUSSION

Our experience and review of literature suggests that the central nervous system of warm-blooded animals and humans seem to work in relatively congruent ways. As such, it can be anticipated that abnormal brain wave patterns like those seen in human cases of aggression, impulsivity, anxiety, depression, epilepsy, head injury, and other clinical conditions are also likely to be found in animals. When this is the case, neurofeedback may have potential to assist the behavioral and brain dysfunctions of animals as well as humans.

The LENS neurofeedback only requires the subject to remain motionless for a few seconds and does not require concentration. Therefore, it seems ideally suited to work with animals and small children. Positive effects are often seen after only a few treatments, although in animals as well as humans, a certain number of repeated treatments seem necessary for the positive improvements to become enduring. Small children and animals are more innocent and free of the various defense mechanisms so common in adults. For this reason we may be able to discern more readily the effects of neurofeedback treatment with these groups. A dog or a horse is not particularly impressed by the fact that just because electrodes are being put on his head that he should feel and behave better.

Admittedly the results of our initial uncontrolled case reports with animals are preliminary, based on a limited sample, and they only involved three species. Nonetheless, we observed positive behavioral changes in all cases. We are encouraged by the initial results and believe that other clinicians, as well as researchers, will find that after only a very small number of LENS treatment sessions that animals with behavioral or brain-related problems will become easier to treat. Wires are less likely to be ripped off or equipment damaged. Clinical experience has suggested that sometimes it might be advisable with highly reactive animals to use photonic stimulation for a couple of sessions prior to LENS treatment to calm them and relieve their pain or irritation. With "fear-biting"

FIGURE 7. Jock and Dog Pre- and Post-Treatment Ratings

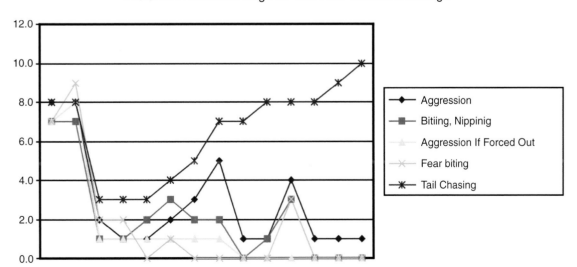

dogs a muzzle might be employed for the safety of the clinician/experimenter. Normally animals must be sedated or rigidly confined (locked into braces or restraints) in order to perform EEGs. Our work is unique in that the animals were awake with sedation only required in one case, and the only restraints consisted of humans gently holding the animals.

The animals in our cases were domestic or farm animals, accustomed to interaction with humans, rather than wild or laboratory subjects. It has clearly been our impression that the problems in these animals have often stemmed from less than ideal treatment by humans, and so it is encouraging to us to find that a therapeutic procedure that evolved for treating humans may also be helpful for animals. All too often animals that are having problems are simply "put down." We are pleased to think that a gentle and relatively rapid treatment such as LENS may improve the quality of life of pets that are often very loved by their owners, and it may give many animals a chance to live.

The nature of the LENS provides a unique opportunity for placebo-controlled, double-blinded research with animals (as well as humans). We hope that future research will include animals of several different species. We believe, as in the case of Gandalf that rescue animals who have suffered from accidents or human abuse, as well as animals with head injuries, in zoos or circuses, and that have problems with aggressiveness or obsessive responses, may be ideal candidates for treatment and research. LENS seems to hold promise offering many of these unfortunate animals a chance for a happier adaptation to their lives with a healthier central nervous system.

REFERENCES

Ayers, M. (1987). Electroencephalographic neurofeedback and closed head injury of 250 individuals. National Head Injury Foundation Syllabus, *Head Injury Frontiers*, 380.

Donaldson, C. C. S., Sella, G. E., & Mueller, H. H. (1998). Fibromyalgia: A retrospective study of 252 consecutive referrals. *Canadian Journal of Clinical Medicine, 5* (6), 116-127.

Egner, T., & Gruzelier, J. H. (2003). Ecological validity of neurofeedback: Modulation of slow wave EEG enhances musical performance. *NeuroReport, 14* (9), 1221-1224.

Egner, T., & Sterman, M. B. (2006). Neurofeedback treatment of epilepsy: From basic rationale to practical application. *Expert Review of Neurotherapeutics, 6* (2), 247-257.

Fernandez, T., Herrera, W., Harmony, T., Diaz-Comas, L., Santiago, E., Sanchez, L. et al. (2003). EEG and behavioral changes following neurofeedback treatment in learning disabled children. *Clinical Electroencephalography, 34* (3), 145-150.

Green, E., & Green, A. (1986). Biofeedback and states of consciousness. In B. B. Wolman & M. Ullman (Eds.), *Handbook of states of consciousness*. New York: Van Nostrand Reinhold.

Green, E., Green, A., & Walters, D. (1970). Voluntary control of internal states: Psychological and physiological. *Journal of Transpersonal Psychology, 11*, 1-26.

Hammond, D. C. (in press). What is neurofeedback? *Journal of Neurotherapy*.

Hammond, D. C. (2005). Neurofeedback with anxiety and affective disorders. *Child and Adolescent Psychiatric Clinics of North America, 14* (1), 105-123.

Holliday, T. A., & Williams, C. (1999). *Clinical encephalography in dogs*. Davis, CA: Veterinary Medical Teaching Hospital and Department of Surgical and Radiological Sciences, University of California Davis. (*www.neurovet.org*)

Holliday, T. A., & Williams, C. (2003). *Advantages of digital electroencephalography in clinical veterinary medicine, 1*. Davis, CA: Veterinary Medical Teaching Hospital and Department of Surgical and Radiological Sciences, University of California Davis. (*www.neurovet.org*)

Larsen, S. (2006). *The healing power of neurofeedback: The revolutionary LENS technique for restoring optimal brain function*. Rochester, VT: Healing Arts Press.

Lubar, J. F. (1977). Use of biofeedback in the treatment of seizure disorders and hyperactivity. In B. B. Lahey & E. E. Kazdin (Eds.), *Advances in child clinical psychology*. New York: Plenum Publishing.

Lubar, J. F. (2003). Neurofeedback for the management of attention-deficit/hyperactivity disorders. Chapter in M. S. Schwartz & F. Andrasik (Eds.), *Biofeedback: A practitioners guide* (3rd ed., pp. 409-437). New York: Guilford.

Miller, N. E. (1969). Learning of visceral and glandular responses. *Science, 163*, 434-445.

Monastra, V. J., Lynn, S., Linden, M., Lubar, J. F., Gruzelier, J., & LaVaque, T. J. (2005). Electroencephalograpic biofeedback in the treatment of attention-deficit/hyperactivity disorder. *Applied Psychophysiology & Biofeedback, 30* (2), 95-114.

Moore, N. C. (2000). A review of EEG biofeedback treatment of anxiety disorders. *Clinical Electroencephalography, 31* (1), 1-6.

Mueller, H. H., Donaldson, C. C. S., Nelson, D. V., & Layman, M. (2001). Treatment of fibromyalgia incorporating EEG-driven stimulation: A clinical outcomes study. *Journal of Clinical Psychology, 57* (7), 933-952.

Ochs, L. (1994). New light on lights, sounds, and the brain. *Megabrain report: The journal of mind technology, 2* (4), 48-52.

Ochs, L. (1996). Thoughts about EEG-driven stimulation after three years of its uses: Ramifications for concepts of pathology, recovery, and brain function. Unpublished manupscript.

Ochs, L. (2006). Low Energy Neurofeedback System (LENS): Theory, background, and introduction. *Journal of Neurotherapy, 10* (2/3), 5-39.

Peniston, E. G., & Kulkosky, P. J. (1991). Alcoholic personality and alpha-theta brainwave training. *Medical Psychotherapy, 2*, 37-55.

Peniston, E. G., Marrinan, D. A., Deming, W. A., & Kulkosky, P. J. (1993). EEG alpha-theta brainwave synchronization in Vietnam theater veterans with combat-related post-traumatic stress disorder and alcohol abuse. *Advances in Medical Psychotherapy, 6*, 37-50.

Raymond, J., Sajid, I., Parkinson, L. A., & Gruzelier, J. H. (2005). Biofeedback and dance performance: A preliminary investigation. *Applied Psychophysiology & Biofeedback, 30* (1), 65-74.

Schoenberger, N. E., Shiflett, S. C., Esty, M. L., Ochs, L. & Matheis, R. J. (2001). Flexyx Neurotherapy System in the treatment of traumatic brain injury: An initial evaluation. *Journal of Head Trauma Rehabilitation, 16* (3), 260-274.

Sterman, M. B. (1977). EEG biofeedback training in the treatment of epilepsy. In S. Padnes & T. Budzynski (Eds.) NC 6 Roche Scientific Series.

Sterman, M. B., & Friar, L. (1971). Suppression of seizures in an epileptic following sensorimotor EEG feedback training. *Electroencephalography and Clinical Neurophysiology, 1*, 57-86.

Sterman, M. B., & Friar, L. (2000). Suppression of seizues in an epileptic following sensorimotor EEG feedback training. *Electroencephalography and Clinical Neurophysiology, 31* (1), 45-55.

doi:10.1300/J184v10n02_08

APPENDIX

CNS Questionnaire for Animals

Name:_____

Rate all relevant items on a scale of 0-10 (10 is the worst possible, 0 means the problem ceases to be relevant)

Cognitive/Mental   **Dates:**

Anticipatory, trying too hard
Ungenerous, miserly with mental effort
Stuck, inability to learn new behaviors
Rigid, inability to unlearn old behaviors
Poor Memory
ADHD or ADD type behaviors
Suspicious

Sensitivity/Reactivity

Startles easily, hypervigilant
Reacts to fly spray
Reacts negatively to washing/brushing

APPENDIX (continued)

Neurological Problems   **Dates:**

Head tilting
Tongue lolling
Anxiety
Depression
Panic attacks, heart pounding
Nervous sweating
Nervous gulping
Restlessness
Overly fearful, phobic
Muscular tension (in jaw, neck, back)

Social Problems

Dominance problem, excessively aggressive
Fear of solitude, exaggerated
Screaming, neighing
Excluded/Rejected other animals
Rough play, Compulsive

Behavioral Problems

Stall walking/Fence pacing
Cribbing, chewing on foreign objects
Eating dirt, manure
Tense, rigid movements
Inability to accept normal handling
Explosive, can't return to normal
Kicking at air
Head bobbing, swinging
Trailering phobia
Biting, nipping

Physiological/Medical Conditions　　　　　　　　　　　**Dates:**

Lethargic, dull

Lyme disease

Primarily Dogs

Aggression to other animals

Aggression to humans

Disobedient

Runs away

Self-mutilation, chewing, scratching

Stubborn, refuses to be trained

Housebreaking problem

Spite soiling to punish owners

Passive/Aggressive

Chases cars

Barking, neurotic

Hides, especially after bad behavior

Aggressive if you force him/her out

Fear biting or sudden biting

Inappropriate rolling-over

Gets into garbage

Gets on furniture, even when scolded

Tail chasing

Primarily Cats

Biting/clawing as play becomes suddenly aggressive

Aggressive to other animals

Aggressive toward people

Spraying inside house

Other housebreaking problem

Overeating, eating too fast, throwing up

Ripping fur out

APPENDIX (continued)

Primarily Cats (continued)   **Dates:**

Jumps on table or other furniture when knowing it's forbidden
Digs claws in while on lap or being petted
Distant, unaffectionate
Excessively affectionate

Index

Page numbers in *italics* designate figures; page numbers followed by "t" designate tables.